The World Health Report **2008**

Primary Health Care

Now More Than Ever

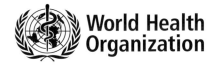

World Health Organization

WHO Library Cataloguing-in-Publication Data

The world health report 2008 : primary health care now more than ever.

1.World health – trends. 2.Primary health care – trends. 3.Delivery of health care. 4.Health policy.
I.World Health Organization.

ISBN 978 92 4 156373 4   (NLM classification: W 84.6)

ISSN 1020-3311

Information concerning this publication can be obtained from:

World Health Report
World Health Organization
1211 Geneva 27, Switzerland
E-mail: whr@who.int

Copies of this publication can be ordered from: bookorders@who.int

The World Health Report 2008 was produced under the overall direction of Tim Evans (Assistant Director-General) and Wim Van Lerberghe (editor-in-chief). The principal writing team consisted of Wim Van Lerberghe, Tim Evans, Kumanan Rasanathan and Abdelhay Mechbal. Other main contributors to the drafting of the report were: Anne Andermann, David Evans, Benedicte Galichet, Alec Irwin, Mary Kay Kindhauser, Remo Meloni, Thierry Mertens, Charles Mock, Hernan Montenegro, Denis Porignon and Dheepa Rajan. Organizational supervision of the report was provided by Ramesh Shademani.

Contributions in the form of boxes, figures and data analysis came from: Alayne Adams, Jonathan Abrahams, Fiifi Amoako Johnson, Giovanni Ancona, Chris Bailey, Robert Beaglehole, Henk Bekedam, Andre Biscaia, Paul Bossyns, Eric Buch, Andrew Cassels, Somnath Chatterji, Mario Dal Poz, Pim De Graaf, Jan De Maeseneer, Nick Drager, Varatharajan Durairaj, Joan Dzenowagis, Dominique Egger, Ricardo Fabregas, Paulo Ferrinho, Daniel Ferrante, Christopher Fitzpatrick, Gauden Galea, Claudia Garcia Moreno, André Griekspoor, Lieve Goeman, Miriam Hirschfeld, Ahmadreza Hosseinpoor, Justine Hsu, Chandika Indikadahena, Mie Inoue, Lori Irwin, Andre Isakov, Michel Jancloes, Miloud Kaddar, Hyppolite Kalambaye, Guy Kegels, Meleckidzedeck Khayesi, Ilona Kickbush, Yohannes Kinfu, Tord Kjellstrom, Rüdiger Krech, Mohamed Laaziri, Colin Mathers, Zoe Matthews, Maureen Mackintosh, Di McIntyre, David Meddings, Pierre Mercenier, Pat Neuwelt, Paolo Piva, Annie Portela, Yongyut Ponsupap, Amit Prasad, Rob Ridley, Ritu Sadana, David Sanders, Salif Samake, Gerard Schmets, Iqbal Shah, Shaoguang Wang, Anand Sivasankara Kurup, Kenji Shibuya, Michel Thieren, Nicole Valentine, Nathalie Van de Maele, Jeanette Vega, Jeremy Veillard and Bob Woollard.

Valuable inputs in the form of contributions, peer reviews, suggestions and criticisms were received from the Regional Directors and their staff, from the Deputy Director-General, Anarfi Asamoah Bah, and from the Assistant Directors-General.

The draft report was peer reviewed at a meeting in Montreux, Switzerland, with the following participants: Azrul Azwar, Tim Evans, Ricardo Fabrega, Sheila Campbell-Forrester, Antonio Duran, Alec Irwin, Mohamed Ali Jaffer, Safurah Jaafar, Pongpisut Jongudomsuk, Joseph Kasonde, Kamran Lankarini, Abdelhay Mechbal, John Martin, Donald Matheson, Jan De Maeseneer, Ravi Narayan, Sydney Saul Ndeki, Adrian Ong, Pongsadhorn Pokpermdee, Thomson Prentice, Kumanan Rasanathan, Salman Rawaf, Bijan Sadrizadeh, Hugo Sanchez, Ramesh Shademani, Barbara Starfield, Than Tun Sein, Wim Van Lerberghe, Olga Zeus and Maria Hamlin Zuniga.

The report benefited greatly from the inputs of the following participants in a one-week workshop in Bellagio, Italy: Ahmed Abdullatif, Chris Bailey, Douglas Bettcher, John Bryant, Tim Evans, Marie Therese Feuerstein, Abdelhay Mechbal, Thierry Mertens, Hernan Montenegro, Ronald Labonte, Socrates Litsios, Thelma Narayan, Thomson Prentice, Kumanan Rasanathan, Myat Htoo Razak, Ramesh Shademani, Viroj Tangcharoensathien, Wim Van Lerberghe, Jeanette Vega and Jeremy Veillard.

WHO working groups provided the initial inputs into the report. These working groups, of both HQ and Regional staff included: Shelly Abdool, Ahmed Abdullatif, Shambhu Acharya, Chris Bailey, James Bartram, Douglas Bettcher, Eric Blas, Ties Boerma, Robert Bos, Marie-Charlotte Boueseau, Gui Carrin, Venkatraman Chandra-Mouli, Yves Chartier, Alessandro Colombo, Carlos Corvalan, Bernadette Daelmans, Denis Daumerie, Tarun Dua, Joan Dzenowagis, David Evans, Tim Evans, Bob Fryatt, Michelle Funk, Chad Gardner, Giuliano Gargioni, Gulin Gedik, Sandy Gove, Kersten Gutschmidt, Alex Kalache, Alim Khan, Ilona Kickbusch, Yunkap Kwankam, Richard Laing, Ornella Lincetto, Daniel Lopez-Acuna, Viviana Mangiaterra, Colin Mathers, Michael Mbizvo, Abdelhay Mechbal, Kamini Mendis, Shanthi Mendis, Susan Mercado, Charles Mock, Hernan Montenegro, Catherine Mulholland, Peju Olukoya, Annie Portela, Thomson Prentice, Annette Pruss-Ustun, Kumanan Rasanathan, Myat Htoo Razak, Lina Tucker Reinders, Elil Renganathan, Gojka Roglic, Michael Ryan, Shekhar Saxena, Robert Scherpbier, Ramesh Shademani, Kenji Shibuya, Sameen Siddiqi, Orielle Solar, Francisco Songane, Claudia Stein, Kwok-Cho Tang, Andreas Ullrich, Mukund Uplekar, Wim Van Lerberghe, Jeanette Vega, Jeremy Veillard, Eugenio Villar, Diana Weil and Juliana Yartey.

The editorial production team was led by Thomson Prentice, managing editor. The report was edited by Diana Hopkins, assisted by Barbara Campanini. Gaël Kernen assisted on graphics and produced the web site version and other electronic media. Lina Tucker Reinders provided editorial advice. The index was prepared by June Morrison.

Administrative support in the preparation of the report was provided by Saba Amdeselassie, Maryse Coutty, Melodie Fadriquela, Evelyne Omukubi and Christine Perry.

Photo credits: Director-General's photograph: WHO (p. viii); introduction and overview: WHO/Marco Kokic (p. x); chapters 1–6: Alayne Adams (p. 1); WHO/Christopher Black (p. 23); WHO/Karen Robinson (p. 41); International Federation of Red Cross and Red Crescent Societies/John Haskew (p. 63); Alayne Adams (p. 81); WHO/Thomas Moran (p. 99).

Design: Reda Sadki
Layout: Steve Ewart and Reda Sadki
Figures: Christophe Grangier
Printing Coordination: Pascale Broisin and Frédérique Robin-Wahlin

Printed in Switzerland

Contents

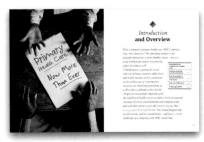

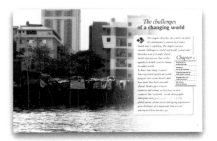

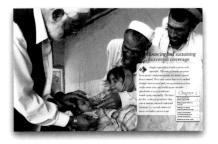

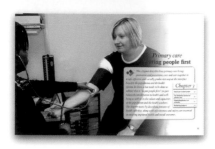

Chapter 3. Primary care: putting people first | 41

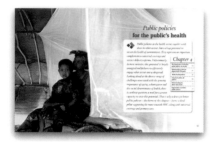

Chapter 4. Public policies for the public's health | 63

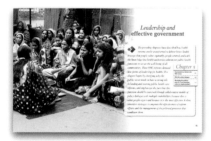

Chapter 5. Leadership and effective government | 81

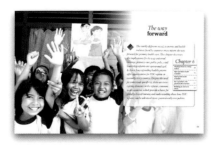

Chapter 6. The way forward | 99

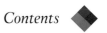
List of Figures

List of Boxes

List of Tables

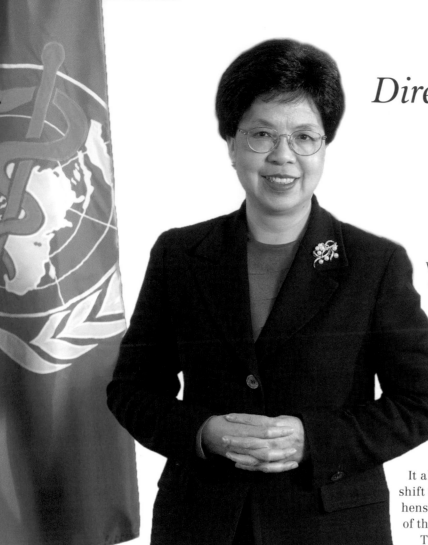

Director-General's **Message**

When I took office in 2007, I made clear my commitment to direct WHO's attention towards primary health care. More important than my own conviction, this reflects the widespread and growing demand for primary health care from Member States. This demand in turn displays a growing appetite among policy-makers for knowledge related to how health systems can become more equitable, inclusive and fair. It also reflects, more fundamentally, a shift towards the need for more compre- hensive thinking about the performance of the health system as a whole.

This year marks both the 60th birth- day of WHO and the 30th anniversary of the Declaration of Alma-Ata on Primary Health Care in 1978. While our global health context has changed remarkably over six decades, the values that lie at the core of the WHO Constitution and those that informed the Alma-Ata Declaration have been tested and remain true. Yet, despite enormous progress in health globally, our collective fail- ures to deliver in line with these values are painfully obvious and deserve our greatest attention.

We see a mother suffering complications of labour without access to qualified support, a child missing out on essential vaccinations, an inner-city slum dweller living in squalor. We see the absence of protection for pedestrians alongside traffic-laden roads and highways, and the impoverishment arising from direct payment for care because of a lack of health insurance. These and many other everyday realities of life personify the unacceptable and avoidable shortfalls in the performance of our health systems.

In moving forward, it is important to learn from the past and, in looking back, it is clear that we can do better in the future. Thus, this World Health Report revisits the ambitious vision of primary health care as a set of values and principles for guiding the development of health systems. The Report represents an important opportunity to draw on the lessons of the past, consider the challenges that lie ahead, and identify major avenues for health systems to narrow the intolerable gaps between aspiration and implementation.

These avenues are defined in the Report as four sets of reforms that reflect a convergence between the values of primary health care, the expectations of citizens and the common health performance challenges that cut across all contexts. They include:

- *universal coverage reforms* that ensure that health systems contribute to health equity, social justice and the end of exclusion, primarily by moving towards universal access and social health protection;
- *service delivery reforms* that re-organize health services around people's needs and expectations, so as to make them more socially relevant and more responsive to the changing world, while producing better outcomes;
- *public policy reforms* that secure healthier communities, by integrating public health actions with primary care, by pursuing healthy public policies across sectors and by strengthening national and transnational public health interventions; and
- *leadership reforms* that replace disproportionate reliance on command and control on one hand, and laissez-faire disengagement of the state on the other, by the inclusive, participatory, negotiation-based leadership indicated by the complexity of contemporary health systems.

While universally applicable, these reforms do not constitute a blueprint or a manifesto for action. The details required to give them life in each country must be driven by specific conditions and contexts, drawing on the best available evidence. Nevertheless, there are no reasons why any country – rich or poor – should wait to begin moving forward with these reforms. As the last three decades have demonstrated, substantial progress is possible.

Doing better in the next 30 years means that we need to invest now in our ability to bring actual performance in line with our aspirations, expectations and the rapidly changing realities of our interdependent health world. United by the common challenge of primary health care, the time is ripe, now more than ever, to foster joint learning and sharing across nations to chart the most direct course towards health for all.

Dr Margaret Chan
Director-General
World Health Organization

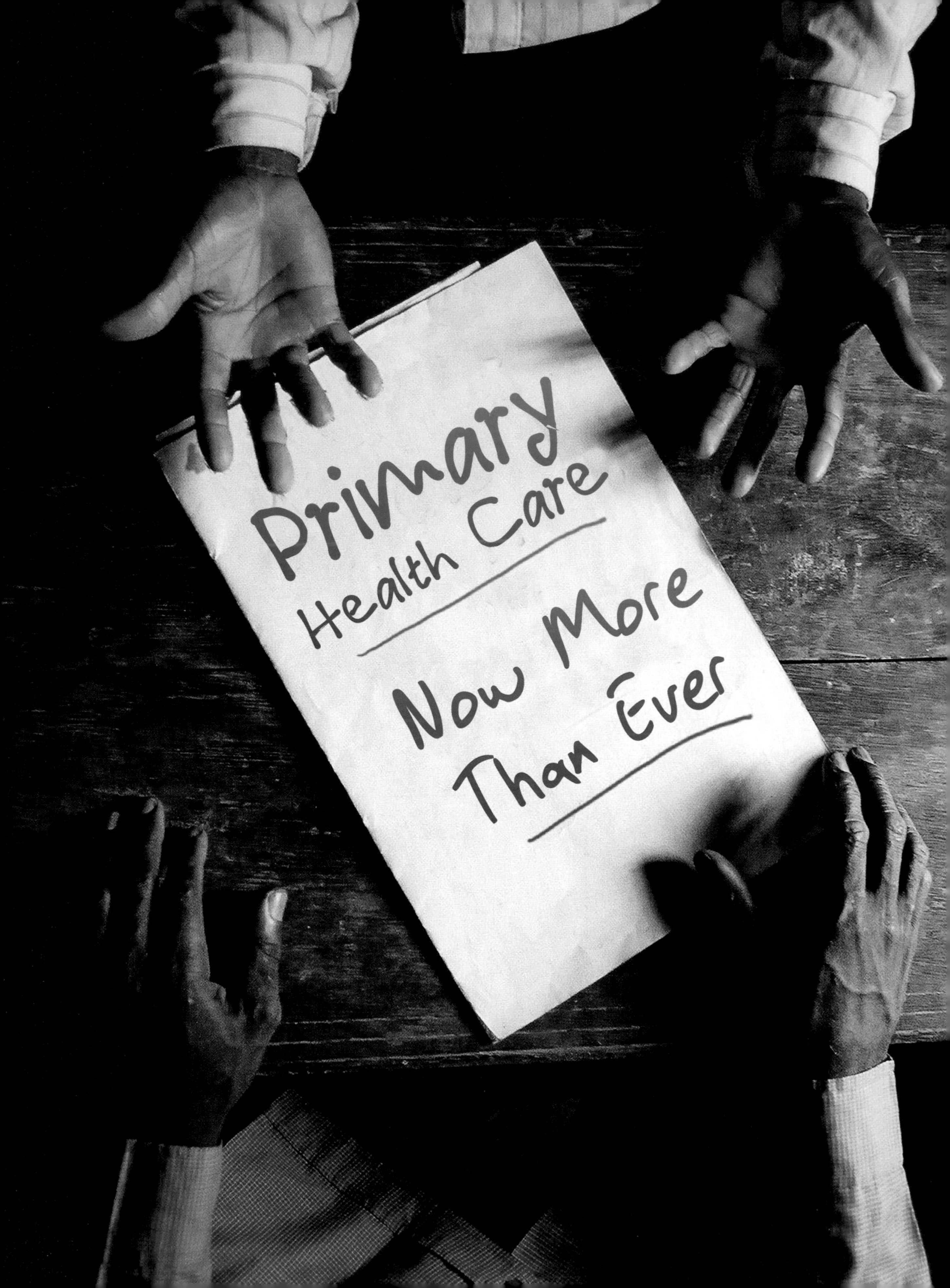
Primary
Health Care
Now More
Than Ever

Introduction
and Overview

Why a renewal of primary health care (PHC), and why now, more than ever? The immediate answer is the palpable demand for it from Member States – not just from health professionals, but from the political arena as well.

Globalization is putting the social cohesion of many countries under stress, and health systems, as key constituents of the architecture of contemporary societies, are clearly not performing as well as they could and as they should.

People are increasingly impatient with the inability of health services to deliver levels of national coverage that meet stated demands and changing needs, and with their failure to provide services in ways that correspond to their expectations. Few would disagree that health systems need to respond better – and faster – to the challenges of a changing world. PHC can do that.

There is today a recognition that populations are left behind and a sense of lost opportunities that are reminiscent of what gave rise, thirty years ago, to Alma-Ata's paradigm shift in thinking about health. The Alma-Ata Conference mobilized a "Primary Health Care movement" of professionals and institutions, governments and civil society organizations, researchers and grassroots organizations that undertook to tackle the "*politically, socially and economically unacceptable*"[1] health inequalities in all countries. The Declaration of Alma-Ata was clear about the values pursued: social justice and the right to better health for all, participation and solidarity[1]. There was a sense that progress towards these values required fundamental changes in the way health-care systems operated and harnessed the potential of other sectors.

The translation of these values into tangible reforms has been uneven. Nevertheless, today, health equity enjoys increased prominence in the discourse of political leaders and ministries of health[2], as well as of local government structures, professional organizations and civil society organizations.

The PHC values to achieve health for all require health systems that "*Put people at the centre of health care*"[3]. What people consider desirable ways of living as individuals and what they expect for their societies – i.e. what people value – constitute important parameters for governing the health sector. PHC has remained the benchmark for most countries' discourse on health precisely because the PHC movement tried to provide rational, evidence-based and anticipatory responses to health needs *and* to these social expectations[4,5,6,7]. Achieving this requires trade-offs that must start by taking into account citizens' "*expectations about health and health care*" and ensuring "*that [their] voice and choice decisively influence the way in which health services are designed and operate*"[8]. A recent PHC review echoes this perspective as the "*right to the highest attainable level of health*", "*maximizing equity and solidarity*" while being guided by "*responsiveness to people's needs*"[4]. Moving towards health for all requires that health systems respond to the challenges of a changing world and growing expectations for better performance. This involves substantial reorientation and reform of the ways health systems operate in society today: those reforms constitute the agenda of the renewal of PHC.

Responding to the challenges of a changing world

On the whole, people are healthier, wealthier and live longer today than 30 years ago. If children were still dying at 1978 rates, there would have been 16.2 million deaths globally in 2006. In fact, there were only 9.5 million such deaths[9]. This difference of 6.7 million is equivalent to 18 329 children's lives being saved every day. The once revolutionary notion of essential drugs has become commonplace. There have been significant improvements in access to water, sanitation and antenatal care.

This shows that progress is possible. It can also be accelerated. There have never been more resources available for health than now. The global health economy is growing faster than gross domestic product (GDP), having increased its share from 8% to 8.6% of the world's GDP between 2000 and 2005. In absolute terms, adjusted for inflation, this represents a 35% growth in the world's expenditure on health over a five-year period. Knowledge and understanding of health are growing rapidly. The accelerated technological revolution is multiplying the potential for improving health and transforming health literacy in a better-educated and modernizing global society. A global stewardship is emerging: from intensified exchanges between countries, often in recognition of shared threats, challenges or opportunities; from growing solidarity; and from the global commitment to eliminate poverty exemplified in the Millennium Development Goals (MDGs).

However, there are other trends that must not be ignored. First, the substantial progress in health over recent decades has been deeply unequal, with convergence towards improved health in a large part of the world, but at the same time, with a considerable number of countries increasingly lagging behind or losing ground. Furthermore, there is now ample documentation – not available 30 years ago – of considerable and often growing health inequalities within countries.

Second, the nature of health problems is changing in ways that were only partially anticipated, and at a rate that was wholly unexpected. Ageing and the effects of ill-managed urbanization and globalization accelerate worldwide transmission of communicable diseases, and increase the burden of chronic and noncommunicable disorders. The growing reality that many individuals present with complex symptoms and multiple illnesses challenges service delivery to develop more integrated and comprehensive case management. A complex web of interrelated factors is at work, involving gradual but long-term increases in income and population, climate change, challenges to food security, and social tensions, all with definite, but largely unpredictable, implications for health in the years ahead.

Third, health systems are not insulated from the rapid pace of change and transformation that is an essential part of today's globalization. Economic and political crises challenge state and institutional roles to ensure access, delivery and financing. Unregulated commercialization is accompanied by a blurring of the boundaries between public and private actors, while the negotiation of entitlement and rights is increasingly politicized. The information age has transformed the relations between citizens, professionals and politicians.

In many regards, the responses of the health sector to the changing world have been inadequate and naïve. Inadequate, insofar as they not only fail to anticipate, but also to respond appropriately: too often with too little, too late or too much in the wrong place. Naïve insofar as a system's failure requires a system's solution – not a temporary remedy. Problems with human resources for public health and health care, finance, infrastructure or information systems invariably extend beyond the narrowly defined health sector, beyond a single level of policy purview and, increasingly, across borders: this raises the benchmark in terms of working effectively across government and stakeholders.

While the health sector remains massively under-resourced in far too many countries, the resource base for health has been growing consistently over the last decade. The opportunities this growth offers for inducing structural changes and making health systems more effective and equitable are often missed. Global and, increasingly, national policy formulation processes have focused on single issues, with various constituencies competing for scarce resources, while scant attention is given to the underlying constraints that hold up health systems development in national contexts. Rather than improving their response capacity and anticipating new challenges, health systems seem to be drifting from one short-term priority to another, increasingly fragmented and without a clear sense of direction.

Today, it is clear that left to their own devices, health systems do not gravitate naturally towards the goals of health for all through primary health care as articulated in the Declaration of Alma-Ata. Health systems are developing in directions that contribute little to equity and social justice and fail to get the best health outcomes for their money. Three particularly worrisome trends can be characterized as follows:

- health systems that focus disproportionately on a narrow offer of specialized curative care;
- health systems where a command-and-control approach to disease control, focused on short-term results, is fragmenting service delivery;
- health systems where a hands-off or laissez-faire approach to governance has allowed unregulated commercialization of health to flourish.

These trends fly in the face of a comprehensive and balanced response to health needs. In a number of countries, the resulting inequitable access, impoverishing costs, and erosion of trust in health care constitute a threat to social stability.

Growing expectations for better performance

The support for a renewal of PHC stems from the growing realization among health policy-makers that it can provide a stronger sense of direction and unity in the current context of fragmentation of health systems, and an alternative to the assorted quick fixes currently touted as cures for the health sector's ills. There is also a growing realization that conventional health-care delivery, through different mechanisms and for different reasons, is not only less effective than it could be, but suffers from a set of ubiquitous shortcomings and contradictions that are summarized in Box 1.

The mismatch between expectations and performance is a cause of concern for health authorities. Given the growing economic weight and social significance of the health sector, it is also an increasing cause for concern among politicians: it is telling that health-care issues were, on average, mentioned more than 28 times in each of the recent primary election debates in the United States[22]. Business as usual for health systems is not a viable option. If these shortfalls in performance are to be redressed, the health

problems of today and tomorrow will require stronger collective management and accountability guided by a clearer sense of overall direction and purpose.

Indeed, this is what people expect to happen. As societies modernize, people demand more from their health systems, for themselves and their families, as well as for the society in which they live. Thus, there is increasingly popular support for better health equity and an end to exclusion; for health services that are centred on people's needs and expectations; for health security for the communities in which they live; and for a say in what affects their health and that of their communities[23].

These expectations resonate with the values that were at the core of the Declaration of Alma-Ata. They explain the current demand for a better alignment of health systems with these values and provide today's PHC movement with reinvigorated social and political backing for its attempts to reform health systems.

From the packages of the past to the reforms of the future

Rising expectations and broad support for the vision set forth in Alma-Ata's values have not always easily translated into effective transformation of health systems. There have been circumstances and trends from beyond the health sector – structural adjustment, for example – over which the PHC movement had little influence or control. Furthermore, all too often, the PHC movement has oversimplified its message, resulting in one-size-fits-all recipes, ill-adapted to different contexts and problems[24]. As a result, national and global health authorities have at times seen PHC not as a set of reforms, as was intended, but as one health-care delivery programme among many, providing poor care for poor people. Table 1 looks at different dimensions of early attempts at implementing PHC and contrasts this with current approaches. Inherent in this evolution is recognition that providing a sense of direction to health systems requires a set of specific and context-sensitive reforms that respond to the health challenges of today and prepare for those of tomorrow.

Box 1 Five common shortcomings of health-care delivery

Inverse care. People with the most means – whose needs for health care are often less – consume the most care, whereas those with the least means and greatest health problems consume the least[10]. Public spending on health services most often benefits the rich more than the poor[11] in high- and low-income countries alike[12,13].

Impoverishing care. Wherever people lack social protection and payment for care is largely out-of-pocket at the point of service, they can be confronted with catastrophic expenses. Over 100 million people annually fall into poverty because they have to pay for health care[14].

Fragmented and fragmenting care. The excessive specialization of health-care providers and the narrow focus of many disease control programmes discourage a holistic approach to the individuals and the families they deal with and do not appreciate the need for continuity in care[15]. Health services for poor and marginalized groups are often highly fragmented and severely under-resourced[16], while development aid often adds to the fragmentation[17].

Unsafe care. Poor system design that is unable to ensure safety and hygiene standards leads to high rates of hospital-acquired infections, along with medication errors and other avoidable adverse effects that are an underestimated cause of death and ill-health[18].

Misdirected care. Resource allocation clusters around curative services at great cost, neglecting the potential of primary prevention and health promotion to prevent up to 70% of the disease burden[19,20]. At the same time, the health sector lacks the expertise to mitigate the adverse effects on health from other sectors and make the most of what these other sectors can contribute to health[21].

The focus of these reforms goes well beyond "basic" service delivery and cuts across the established boundaries of the building blocks of national health systems[25]. For example, aligning health systems based on the values that drive PHC will require ambitious human resources policies. However, it would be an illusion to think that these can be developed in isolation from financing or service delivery policies, civil service reform and arrangements dealing with the cross-border migration of health professionals.

At the same time, PHC reforms, and the PHC movement that promotes them, have to be more responsive to social change and rising expectations that come with development and modernization. People all over the world are becoming more vocal about health as an integral part of how they and their families go about their everyday lives, and about the way their society deals with health and health care. The dynamics of demand must find a voice within the policy and decision-making processes. The necessary reorientation of health systems has to be based on sound scientific evidence and on rational management of uncertainty, but it should also integrate what people expect of health and health care for themselves, their families and their society. This requires delicate trade-offs and negotiation with multiple stakeholders that imply a stark departure from the linear, top-down models of the past. Thus, PHC reforms today are neither primarily defined by the component elements they address, nor merely by the choice of disease control interventions to be scaled up, but by the social dynamics that define the role of health systems in society.

Table 1 How experience has shifted the focus of the PHC movement

EARLY ATTEMPTS AT IMPLEMENTING PHC	CURRENT CONCERNS OF PHC REFORMS
Extended access to a basic package of health interventions and essential drugs for the rural poor	Transformation and regulation of existing health systems, aiming for universal access and social health protection
Concentration on mother and child health	Dealing with the health of everyone in the community
Focus on a small number of selected diseases, primarily infectious and acute	A comprehensive response to people's expectations and needs, spanning the range of risks and illnesses
Improvement of hygiene, water, sanitation and health education at village level	Promotion of healthier lifestyles and mitigation of the health effects of social and environmental hazards
Simple technology for volunteer, non-professional community health workers	Teams of health workers facilitating access to and appropriate use of technology and medicines
Participation as the mobilization of local resources and health-centre management through local health committees	Institutionalized participation of civil society in policy dialogue and accountability mechanisms
Government-funded and delivered services with a centralized top-down management	Pluralistic health systems operating in a globalized context
Management of growing scarcity and downsizing	Guiding the growth of resources for health towards universal coverage
Bilateral aid and technical assistance	Global solidarity and joint learning
Primary care as the antithesis of the hospital	Primary care as coordinator of a comprehensive response at all levels
PHC is cheap and requires only a modest investment	PHC is not cheap: it requires considerable investment, but it provides better value for money than its alternatives

Four sets of PHC reforms

This report structures the PHC reforms in four groups that reflect the convergence between the evidence on what is needed for an effective response to the health challenges of today's world, the values of equity, solidarity and social justice that drive the PHC movement, and the growing expectations of the population in modernizing societies (Figure 1):

- reforms that ensure that health systems contribute to health equity, social justice and the end of exclusion, primarily by moving towards universal access and social health protection – *universal coverage reforms*;
- reforms that reorganize health services as primary care, i.e. around people's needs and expectations, so as to make them more socially relevant and more responsive to the changing world while producing better outcomes – *service delivery reforms*;
- reforms that secure healthier communities, by integrating public health actions with primary care and by pursuing healthy public policies across sectors – *public policy reforms*;
- reforms that replace disproportionate reliance on command and control on one hand, and laissez-faire disengagement of the state on the other, by the inclusive, participatory, negotiation-based leadership required by the complexity of contemporary health systems – *leadership reforms*.

The first of these four sets of reforms aims at diminishing exclusion and social disparities in health. Ultimately, the determinants of health inequality require a societal response, with political and technical choices that affect many different sectors. Health inequalities are also shaped by the inequalities in availability, access and quality of services, by the financial burden these impose on people, and even by the linguistic, cultural and gender-based barriers that are often embedded in the way in which clinical practice is conducted[26].

If health systems are to reduce health inequities, a precondition is to make services available to all, i.e. to bridge the gap in the supply of services. Service networks are much more extensive today

Figure 1 The PHC reforms necessary to refocus health systems towards health for all

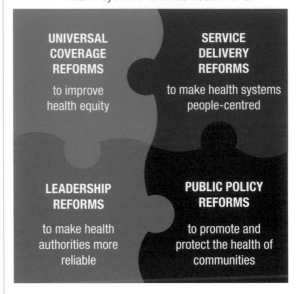

than they were 30 years ago, but large population groups have been left behind. In some places, war and civil strife have destroyed infrastructure, in others, unregulated commercialization has made services available, but not necessarily those that are needed. Supply gaps are still a reality in many countries, making extension of their service networks a priority concern, as was the case 30 years ago.

As the overall supply of health services has improved, it has become more obvious that barriers to access are important factors of inequity: user fees, in particular, are important sources of exclusion from needed care. Moreover, when people have to purchase health care at a price that is beyond their means, a health problem can quickly precipitate them into poverty or bankruptcy[14]. That is why extension of the supply of services has to go hand-in-hand with social health protection, through pooling and pre-payment instead of out-of-pocket payment of user fees. The reforms to bring about universal coverage – i.e. universal access combined with social health protection – constitute a necessary condition to improved health equity. As systems that have achieved near universal coverage show, such reforms need to be complemented with another set of proactive measures to reach the unreached: those for whom service availability and social protection does too little to offset the health consequences of social stratification. Many individuals in this group rely on health-care networks that assume the responsibility for the health of entire communities. This is where a second set of reforms, the service delivery reforms, comes in.

These service delivery reforms are meant to transform conventional health-care delivery into primary care, optimizing the contribution of health services – local health systems, health-care networks, health districts – to health and equity while responding to the growing expectations for *"putting people at the centre of health care, harmonizing mind and body, people and systems"*[3]. These service delivery reforms are but one subset of PHC reforms, but one with such a high profile that it has often masked the broader PHC agenda. The resulting confusion has been compounded by the oversimplification of what primary care entails and of what distinguishes it from conventional health-care delivery (Box 2)[24].

There is a substantial body of evidence on the comparative advantages, in terms of effectiveness and efficiency, of health care organized as people-centred primary care. Despite variations in the specific terminology, its characteristic features (person-centredness, comprehensiveness and integration, continuity of care, and participation of patients, families and communities) are well identified[15,27]. Care that exhibits these features requires health services that are organized accordingly, with close-to-client multidisciplinary teams that are responsible for a defined population, collaborate with social services and other sectors, and coordinate the contributions of hospitals, specialists and community organizations. Recent economic growth has brought additional resources to health. Combined with the growing demand for better performance, this creates major opportunities to reorient existing health services towards primary care – not only in well-resourced settings, but also where money is tight and needs are high. In the many low- and middle-income countries where the supply of services is in a phase of accelerated expansion, there is an opportunity now to chart a course that may avoid repeating some of the mistakes high-income countries have made in the past.

Primary care can do much to improve the health of communities, but it is not sufficient to respond to people's desires to live in conditions that protect their health, support health equity

---

Box 2 What has been considered primary care in well-resourced contexts has been dangerously oversimplified in resource-constrained settings

Primary care has been defined, described and studied extensively in well-resourced contexts, often with reference to physicians with a specialization in family medicine or general practice. These descriptions provide a far more ambitious agenda than the unacceptably restrictive and off-putting primary-care recipes that have been touted for low-income countries[27,28]:

■ primary care provides a place to which people can bring a wide range of health problems – it is not acceptable that in low-income countries primary care would only deal with a few "priority diseases";

■ primary care is a hub from which patients are guided through the health system – it is not acceptable that, in low-income countries, primary care would be reduced to a stand-alone health post or isolated community-health worker;

■ primary care facilitates ongoing relationships between patients and clinicians, within which patients participate in decision-making about their health and health care; it builds bridges between personal health care and patients' families and communities – it is not acceptable that, in low-income countries, primary care would be restricted to a one-way delivery channel for priority health interventions;

■ primary care opens opportunities for disease prevention and health promotion as well as early detection of disease – it is not acceptable that, in low-income countries, primary care would just be about treating common ailments;

■ primary care requires teams of health professionals: physicians, nurse practitioners, and assistants with specific and sophisticated biomedical and social skills – it is not acceptable that, in low-income countries, primary care would be synonymous with low-tech, non-professional care for the rural poor who cannot afford any better;

■ primary care requires adequate resources and investment, and can then provide much better value for money than its alternatives – it is not acceptable that, in low-income countries, primary care would have to be financed through out-of-pocket payments on the erroneous assumption that it is cheap and the poor should be able to afford it.

and enable them to lead the lives that they value. People also expect their governments to put into place an array of public policies to deal with health challenges, such as those posed by urbanization, climate change, gender discrimination or social stratification.

These public policies encompass the technical policies and programmes dealing with priority health problems. These programmes can be designed to work through, support and give a boost to primary care, or they can neglect to do this and, however unwillingly, undermine efforts to reform service delivery. Health authorities have a major responsibility to make the right design decisions. Programmes to target priority health problems through primary care need to be complemented by public-health interventions at national or international level. These may offer scale efficiencies; for some problems, they may be the only workable option. The evidence is overwhelming that action on that scale, for selected interventions, which may range from public hygiene and disease prevention to health promotion, can have a major contribution to health. Yet, they are surprisingly neglected, across all countries, regardless of income level. This is particularly visible at moments of crisis and acute threats to the public's health, when rapid response capacity is essential not only to secure health, but also to maintain the public trust in the health system.

Public policy-making, however, is about more than classical public health. Primary care and social protection reforms critically depend on choosing health-systems policies, such as those related to essential drugs, technology, human resources and financing, which are supportive of the reforms that promote equity and people-centred care. Furthermore, it is clear that population health can be improved through policies that are controlled by sectors other than health. School curricula, the industry's policy towards gender equality, the safety of food and consumer goods, or the transport of toxic waste are all issues that can profoundly influence or even determine the health of entire communities, positively or negatively, depending on what choices are made. With deliberate efforts towards intersectoral collaboration, it is possible to give due consideration to "health in all policies"[29] to ensure that, along with the other sectors' goals and objectives, health effects play a role in public policy decisions.

In order to bring about such reforms in the extraordinarily complex environment of the health sector, it will be necessary to reinvest in public leadership in a way that pursues collaborative models of policy dialogue with multiple stakeholders – because this is what people expect, and because this is what works best. Health authorities can do a much better job of formulating and implementing PHC reforms adapted to specific national contexts and constraints if the mobilization around PHC is informed by the lessons of past successes and failures. The governance of health is a major challenge for ministries of health and the other institutions, governmental and nongovernmental, that provide health leadership. They can no longer be content with mere administration of the system: they have to become learning organizations. This requires inclusive leadership that engages with a variety of stakeholders beyond the boundaries of the public sector, from clinicians to civil society, and from communities to researchers and academia. Strategic areas for investment to improve the capacity of health authorities to lead PHC reforms include making health information systems instrumental to reform; harnessing the innovations in the health sector and the related dynamics in all societies; and building capacity through exchange and exposure to the experience of others – within and across borders.

Seizing opportunities

These four sets of PHC reforms are driven by shared values that enjoy large support and challenges that are common to a globalizing world. Yet, the starkly different realities faced by individual countries must inform the way they are taken forward. The operationalization of universal coverage, service delivery, public policy and leadership reforms cannot be implemented as a blueprint or as a standardized package.

In high-expenditure health economies, which is the case of most high-income countries, there is ample financial room to accelerate the shift from tertiary to primary care, create a healthier policy environment and complement a well-established universal coverage system with targeted measures to reduce exclusion. In the large number of fast-growing health economies – which is where 3 billion people live – that very growth provides opportunities to base health systems on sound primary care and universal coverage principles at a stage where it is in full expansion, avoiding the errors by omission, such as failing to invest in healthy public policies, and by commission, such as investing disproportionately in tertiary care, that have characterized health systems in high-income countries in the recent past. The challenge is, admittedly, more daunting for the 2 billion people living in the low-growth health economies of Africa and South-East Asia, as well as for the more than 500 million who live in fragile states. Yet, even here, there are signs of growth – and evidence of a potential to accelerate it through other means than through the counter-productive reliance on inequitable out-of-pocket payments at points of delivery – that offer possibilities to expand health systems and services. Indeed, more than in other countries, they cannot afford not to opt for PHC and, as elsewhere, they can start doing so right away.

The current international environment is favourable to a renewal of PHC. Global health is receiving unprecedented attention, with growing interest in united action, greater calls for comprehensive and universal care – be it from people living with HIV and those concerned with providing treatment and care, ministers of health, or the Group of Eight (G8) – and a mushrooming of innovative global funding mechanisms related to global solidarity. There are clear and welcome signs of a desire to work together in building sustainable systems for health rather than relying on fragmented and piecemeal approaches[30].

At the same time, there is a perspective of enhanced domestic investment in re-invigorating the health systems around PHC values. The growth in GDP – admittedly vulnerable to economic slowdown, food and energy crises and global warming – is fuelling health spending throughout the world, with the notable exception of fragile states. Harnessing this economic growth would offer opportunities to effectuate necessary PHC reforms that were unavailable during the 1980s and 1990s. Only a fraction of health spending currently goes to correcting common distortions in the way health systems function or to overcoming system bottlenecks that constrain service delivery, but the potential is there and is growing fast.

Global solidarity – and aid – will remain important to supplement and suppport countries making slow progress, but it will become less important per se than exchange, joint learning and global governance. This transition has already taken place in most of the world: most developing countries are *not* aid-dependent. International cooperation can accelerate the conversion of the world's health systems, including through better channelling of aid, but real progress will come from better health governance in countries – low- and high-income alike.

The health authorities and political leaders are ill at ease with current trends in the development of health systems and with the obvious need to adapt to the changing health challenges, demands and rising expectations. This is shaping the current opportunity to implement PHC reforms. People's frustration and pressure for different, more equitable health care and for better health protection for society is building up: never before have expectations been so high about what health authorities and, specifically, ministries of health should be doing about this.

By capitalizing on this momentum, investment in PHC reforms can accelerate the transformation of health systems so as to yield better and more equitably distributed health outcomes. The world has better technology and better information to allow it to maximize the return on transforming the functioning of health systems. Growing civil society involvement in health and scale-efficient collective global thinking (for example, in essential drugs) further contributes to the chances of success.

During the last decade, the global community started to deal with poverty and inequality across the world in a much more systematic way – by setting the MDGs and bringing the issue of inequality to the core of social policy-making. Throughout, health has been a central, closely interlinked concern. This offers opportunities for more effective health action. It also creates the necessary social conditions for the establishment of close alliances beyond the health sector. Thus, intersectoral action is back on centre stage. Many among today's health authorities no longer see their responsibility for health as being limited to survival and disease control, but as one of the key capabilities people and societies value[31].

The legitimacy of health authorities increasingly depends on how well they assume responsibility to develop and reform the health sector according to what people value – in terms of health and of what is expected of health systems in society.

References

1. *Primary health care: report of the International Conference on Primary Health Care, Alma-Ata, USSR, 6–12 September, 1978, jointly sponsored by the World Health Organization and the United Nations Children's Fund.* Geneva, World Health Organization, 1978 (Health for All Series No. 1).

2. Dahlgren G, Whitehead M. Levelling up (part 2): a *discussion paper on European strategies for tackling social inequities in health.* Copenhagen, World Health Organization Regional Office for Europe, 2006 (Studies on social and economic determinants of population health No. 3).

3. WHO Regional Office for South-East Asia and WHO Regional Office for the Western Pacific. *People at the centre of health care: harmonizing mind and body, people and systems.* Geneva, World Health Organization, 2007.

4. *Renewing primary health care in the Americas: a position paper of the Pan American Health Organization.* Washington DC, Pan American Health Organization, 2007.

5. Saltman R, Rico A, Boerma W. *Primary health care in the driver's seat: organizational reform in European primary care.* Maidenhead, England, Open University Press, 2006 (European Observatory on Health Systems and Policies Series).

6. *Report on the review of primary care in the African Region.* Brazzaville, World Health Organization Regional Office for Africa, 2003.

7. *International Conference on Primary Health Care, Alma-Ata: twenty-fifth anniversary.* Geneva, World Health Organization, 2003 (Fifty-sixth World Health Assembly, Geneva, 19–28 May 2003, WHA56.6, Agenda Item 14.18).

8. *The Ljubljana Charter on Reforming Health Care, 1996.* Copenhagen, World Health Organization Regional Office for Europe, 1996.

9. *World Health Statistics 2008.* Geneva, World Health Organization, 2008.

10. Hart T. The inverse care law. *Lancet,* 1971, 1:405–412.

11. *World development report 2004: making services work for poor people.* Washington DC, The World Bank, 2003.

12. Filmer D. *The incidence of public expenditures on health and education.* Washington DC, The World Bank, 2003 (background note for *World development report 2004 – making services work for poor people*).

13. Hanratty B, Zhang T, Whitehead M. How close have universal health systems come to achieving equity in use of curative services? A systematic review. *International Journal of Health Services,* 2007, 37:89–109.

14. Xu K et al. Protecting households from catastrophic health expenditures. *Health Affairs,* 2007, 6:972–983.

15. Starfield B. Policy relevant determinants of health: an international perspective. *Health Policy,* 2002, 60:201–218.

16. Moore G, Showstack J. Primary care medicine in crisis: towards reconstruction and renewal. *Annals of Internal Medicine,* 2003, 138:244–247.

17. Shiffman J. Has donor prioritization of HIV/AIDS displaced aid for other health issues? *Health Policy and Planning,* 2008, 23:95–100.

18. Kohn LT, Corrigan JM, Donaldson MS, eds. *To err is human: building a safer health system.* Washington DC, National Academy Press, Committee on Quality of Care in America, Institute of Medicine, 1999.

19. Fries JF et al. Reducing health care costs by reducing the need and demand for medical services. *New England Journal of Medicine,* 1993, 329:321–325.

20. *The World Health Report 2002 – Reducing risks, promoting healthy life.* Geneva, World Health Organization, 2002.

21. Sindall C. Intersectoral collaboration: the best of times, the worst of times. *Health Promotion International,* 1997, 12(1):5–6.

22. Stevenson D. Planning for the future – long term care and the 2008 election. *New England Journal of Medicine,* 2008, 358:19.

23. Blendon RJ et al. Inequities in health care: a five-country survey. *Health Affairs,* 2002, 21:182–191.

24. Tarimo E, Webster EG. *Primary health care concepts and challenges in a changing world: Alma-Ata revisited.* Geneva, World Health Organization, 1997 (Current concerns ARA paper No. 7).

25. *Everybody's business: strengthening health systems to improve health outcomes: WHO's framework for action.* Geneva, World Health Organization, 2007.

26. Dans A et al. Assessing equity in clinical practice guidelines. *Journal of Clinical Epidemiology,* 2007, 60:540–546.

27. *Primary care. America's health in a new era.* Washington DC, National Academy Press, Institute of Medicine 1996.

28. Starfield B. *Primary care: balancing health needs, services, and technology.* New York, Oxford University Press, 1998.

29. Ståhl T et al, eds. *Health in all policies. Prospects and potentials.* Oslo, Ministry of Social Affairs and Health, 2006.

30. *The Paris declaration on aid effectiveness: ownership, harmonisation, alignment, results and mutual accountability.* Paris, Organisation for Economic Co-operation and Development, 2005.

31. Nussbaum MC, Sen A, eds. *The quality of life.* Oxford, Clarendon Press, 1993.

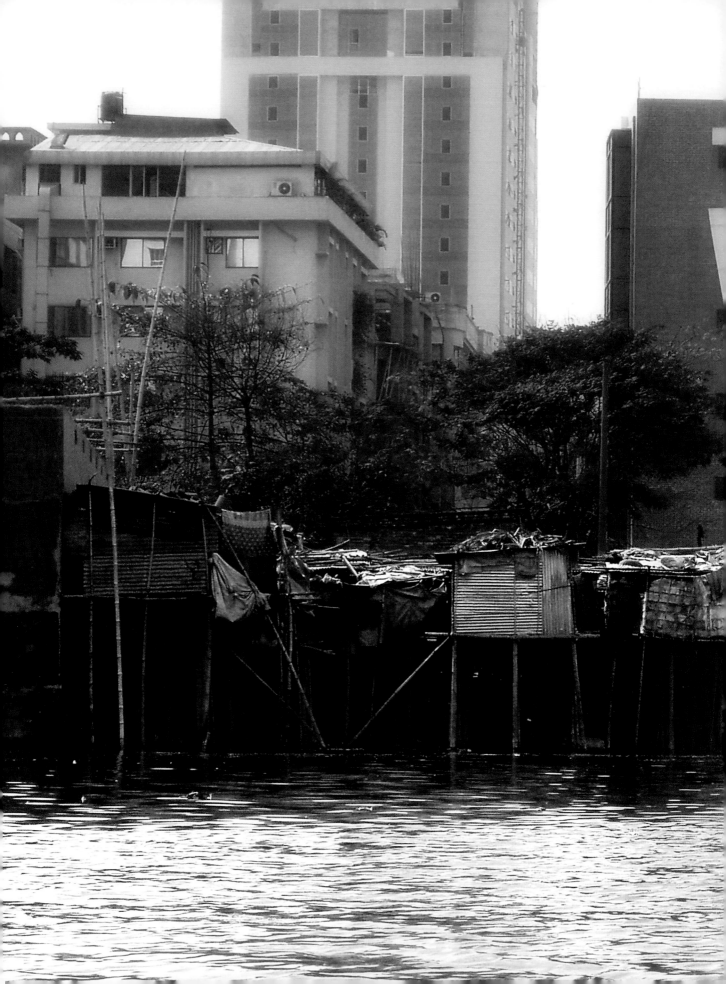

The challenges
of a changing world

This chapter describes the context in which the contemporary renewal of primary health care is unfolding. The chapter reviews current challenges to health and health systems and describes a set of broadly shared social expectations that set the agenda for health systems change in today's world.

It shows how many countries have registered significant health progress over recent decades and how gains have been unevenly shared. Health gaps between countries and among social groups within countries have widened. Social, demographic and epidemiological transformations fed by globalization, urbanization and ageing populations, pose challenges of a magnitude that was not anticipated three decades ago.

The chapter argues that, in general, the response of the health sector and societies to these challenges has been slow and inadequate. This reflects both an inability to mobilize the requisite resources and institutions to transform health around the values of primary health care as well as a failure to either counter or substantially modify forces that pull the health sector in other directions, namely: a disproportionate focus on specialist hospital care; fragmentation of health systems; and the proliferation of unregulated commercial care. Ironically, these powerful trends lead health systems away from what people expect from health and health care. When the Declaration of Alma-Ata enshrined the principles of health equity, people-centred care and a central role for communities in health action, they were considered radical. Social research suggests, however, that these values are becoming mainstream in modernizing societies: they correspond to the way people look at health and what they expect from their health systems. Rising social expectations regarding health and health care, therefore, must be seen as a major driver of PHC reforms.

Unequal growth, unequal outcomes

Longer lives and better health, but not everywhere

In the late 1970s, the Sultanate of Oman had only a handful of health professionals. People had to travel up to four days just to reach a hospital, where hundreds of patients would already be waiting in line to see one of the few (expatriate) doctors. All this changed in less than a generation[1]. Oman invested consistently in a national health service and sustained that investment over time. There is now a dense network of 180 local, district and regional health facilities staffed by over 5000 health workers providing almost universal access to health care for Oman's 2.2 million citizens, with coverage now being extended to foreign residents[2]. Over 98% of births in Oman are now attended by trained personnel and over 98% of infants are fully immunized. Life expectancy at birth, which was less than 60 years towards the end of the 1970s, now surpasses 74 years.

The under-five mortality rate has dropped by a staggering 94%[3].

In each region (except in the African region) there are countries where mortality rates are now less than one fifth of what they were 30 years ago. Leading examples are Chile[4], Malaysia[5], Portugal[6] and Thailand[7] (Figure 1.1). These results were associated with improved access to expanded health-care networks, made possible by sustained political commitment and by economic growth that allowed them to back up their commitment by maintaining investment in the health sector (Box 1.1).

Figure 1.1 Selected best performing countries in reducing under-five mortality by at least 80%, by regions, 1975–2006[a],[*]

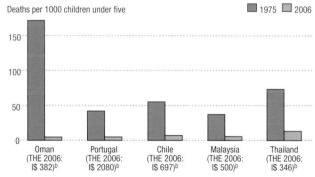

a No country in the African region achieved an 80% reduction.
b Total health expenditure per capita 2006, international $.
* International dollars are derived by dividing local currency units by an estimate of their purchasing power parity compared to the US dollar.

Overall, progress in the world has been considerable. If children were still dying at 1978 rates, there would have been 16.2 million deaths globally in 2006. In fact, there were only 9.5 million such deaths[12]. This difference of 6.7 million is equivalent to 18 329 children's lives being saved every day.

But these figures mask significant variations across countries. Since 1975, the rate of decline in under-five mortality rates has been much slower in low-income countries as a whole than in the richer countries[13]. Apart from Eritrea and Mongolia, none of today's low-income countries has reduced under-five mortality by as much as 70%. The countries that make up today's middle-income countries have done better, but, as Figure 1.3 illustrates, progress has been quite uneven.

Box 1.1 Economic development and investment choices in health care: the improvement of key health indicators in Portugal

Portugal recognized the right to health in its 1976 Constitution, following its democratic revolution. Political pressure to reduce large health inequalities within the country led to the creation of a national health system, funded by taxation and complemented by public and private insurance schemes and out-of-pocket payments[8,9]. The system was fully established between 1979 and 1983 and explicitly organized around PHC principles: a network of health centres staffed by family physicians and nurses progressively covered the entire country. Eligibility for benefits under the national health system requires patients to register with a family physician in a health centre as the first point of contact. Portugal considers this network to be its greatest success in terms of improved access to care and health gains[6].

Life expectancy at birth is now 9.2 years more than it was 30 years ago, while the GDP per capita has doubled. Portugal's performance in reducing mortality in various age groups has been among the world's most consistently successful over the last 30 years, for example halving infant mortality rates every eight years. This performance has led to a marked convergence of the health of Portugal's population with that of other countries in the region[10].

Multivariate analysis of the time series of the various mortality indices since 1960 shows that the decision to base Portugal's health policy on PHC principles, with the development of a network of comprehensive primary care services[11], has played a major role in the reduction of maternal and child mortality, whereas the reduction of perinatal mortality was linked to the development of the hospital network. The relative roles of the development of primary care, hospital networks and economic growth to the improvement of mortality indices since 1960 are shown in Figure 1.2.

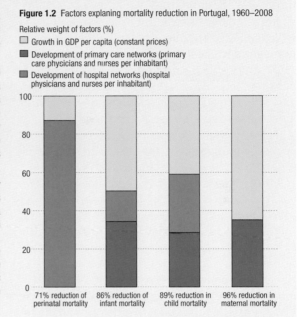

Figure 1.2 Factors explaining mortality reduction in Portugal, 1960–2008

Relative weight of factors (%)
- ☐ Growth in GDP per capita (constant prices)
- ■ Development of primary care networks (primary care physicians and nurses per inhabitant)
- ■ Development of hospital networks (hospital physicians and nurses per inhabitant)

71% reduction of perinatal mortality | 86% reduction of infant mortality | 89% reduction in child mortality | 96% reduction in maternal mortality

Some countries have made great improvements and are on track to achieve the health-related MDGs. Others, particularly in the African region, have stagnated or even lost ground[14]. Globally, 20 of the 25 countries where under-five mortality is still two thirds or more of the 1975 level

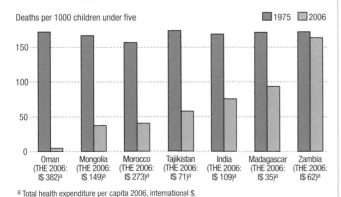

Figure 1.3 Variable progress in reducing under-five mortality, 1975 and 2006, in selected countries with similar rates in 1975[a]

Deaths per 1000 children under five ■ 1975 ■ 2006

Oman (THE 2006: I$ 382)[a] | Mongolia (THE 2006: I$ 149)[a] | Morocco (THE 2006: I$ 273)[a] | Tajikistan (THE 2006: I$ 71)[a] | India (THE 2006: I$ 109)[a] | Madagascar (THE 2006: I$ 35)[a] | Zambia (THE 2006: I$ 62)[a]

a Total health expenditure per capita 2006, international $.

are in sub-Saharan Africa. Slow progress has been associated with disappointing advances in access to health care. Despite recent change for the better, vaccination coverage in sub-Saharan Africa is still significantly lower than in the rest of the world[14]. Current contraceptive prevalence remains as low as 21%, while in other developing regions increases have been substantial over the past 30 years and now reach 61%[15,16]. Increased contraceptive use has been accompanied by decreased abortion rates everywhere. In sub-Saharan Africa, however, the absolute numbers of abortions has increased, and almost all are being performed in unsafe conditions[17]. Childbirth care for mothers and newborns also continues to face problems: in 33 countries, less than half of all births each year are attended by skilled health personnel, with coverage in one country as low as 6%[14]. Sub-Saharan Africa is also the only region in the world where access to qualified providers at childbirth is not progressing[18].

Mirroring the overall trends in child survival, global trends in life expectancy point to a rise throughout the world of almost eight years between 1950 and 1978, and seven more years since: a reflection of the growth in average income per capita. As with child survival, widening income inequality (income increases faster in high-income than in low-income countries) is reflected in increasing disparities between the least and most healthy[19]. Between the mid-1970s and 2005, the difference in life expectancy between high-income countries and countries in sub-Saharan Africa, or fragile states, has widened by 3.8 and 2.1 years, respectively.

The unmistakable relation between health and wealth, summarized in the classic Preston curve (Figure 1.4), needs to be qualified[20].

Firstly, the Preston curve continues to shift[12]. An income per capita of I$ 1000 in 1975 was associated with a life expectancy of 48.8 years. In 2005, it was almost four years higher for the same income. This suggests that improvements in nutrition, education[21], health technologies[22], the institutional capacity to obtain and use information, and in society's ability to translate this knowledge into effective health and social action[23], allow for greater production of health for the same level of wealth.

Figure 1.4 GDP per capita and life expectancy at birth in 169 countries[a], 1975 and 2005

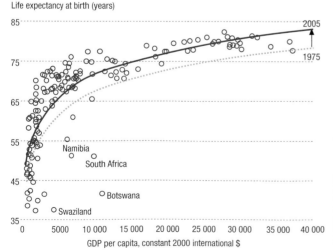

a Only outlying countries are named.

Secondly, there is considerable variation in achievement across countries with the same income, particularly among poorer countries. For example, life expectancy in Côte d'Ivoire (GDP I$ 1465) is nearly 17 years lower than in Nepal (GDP I$ 1379), and between Madagascar and Zambia, the difference is 18 years. The presence of high performers in each income band shows that the actual level of income per capita at a given moment is not the absolute rate limiting factor the average curve seems to imply.

Growth and stagnation

Over the last 30 years the relation between economic growth and life expectancy at birth has shown three distinct patterns (Figure 1.5).

In 1978, about two thirds of the world's population lived in countries that went on to experience increases in life expectancy at birth and considerable economic growth. The most impressive relative gains were in a number of low-income countries in Asia (including India), Latin America and northern Africa, totalling 1.1 billion inhabitants 30 years ago and nearly 2 billion today. These countries increased life expectancy at birth by 12 years, while GDP per capita was multiplied by a factor of 2.6. High-income countries and countries with a GDP between I$ 3000 and I$ 10 000 in 1975 also saw substantial economic growth and increased life expectancy.

In other parts of the world, GDP growth was not accompanied by similar gains in life expectancy. The Russian Federation and Newly Independent States increased average GDP per capita substantially, but, with the widespread poverty that accompanied the transition from the former Soviet Union, women's life expectancy stagnated from the late 1980s and men's plummeted, particularly for those lacking education and job security[24,25]. After a period of technological and organizational stagnation, the health system collapsed[12]. Public expenditure on health declined in the 1990s to levels that made running a basic system virtually impossible in several countries. Unhealthy lifestyles, combined with the disintegration of public health programmes, and the unregulated commercialization of clinical services combined with the elimination of safety nets has offset any gains from the increase in average GDP[26]. China had already increased its

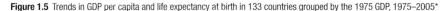

Figure 1.5 Trends in GDP per capita and life expectancy at birth in 133 countries grouped by the 1975 GDP, 1975–2005*

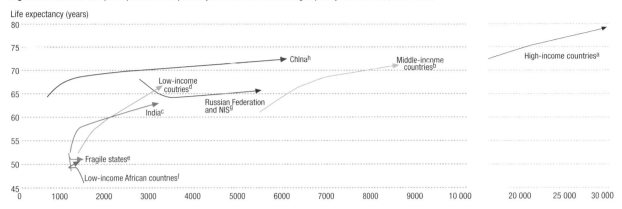

a 27 countries, 766 million (M) inhabitants in 1975, 953 M in 2005.

b 43 countries, 587 M inhabitants in 1975, 986 M in 2005 .

c India, 621 M inhabitants in 1975, 1 103 M in 2005.

d 17 Low-income countries, non-African, fragile states excluded, 471 M inhabitants in 1975, 872 M in 2005.

e 20 Fragile states, 169 M inhabitants in 1975, 374 M in 2005.

f 13 Low-income African countries, fragile states excluded, 71 M inhabitants in 1975, 872 M in 2005.

g Russian Federation and 10 Newly Independent States (NIS), 186 M inhabitants in 1985, 204 M in 2005.

h China, 928 M inhabitants in 1975, 1 316 M in 2005.

* No data for 1975 for the Newly Independant States. No historical data for the remaining countries.

Sources: Life expectancy, 1975, 1985: UN World Population Prospects 2006; 1995, 2005: WHO, 9 November 2008 (draft); China: 3rd, 4th and 5th National Population censuses, 1981, 1990 and 2000. GPD: 2007[37].

life expectancy substantially in the period before 1980 to levels far above that of other low-income countries in the 1970s, despite the 1961–1963 famine and the 1966–1976 Cultural Revolution. The contribution of rural primary care and urban health insurance to this has been well documented[27,28]. With the economic reforms of the early 1980s, however, average GDP per capita increased spectacularly, but access to care and social protection deteriorated, particularly in rural areas. This slowed down improvements to a modest rate, suggesting that only the improved living conditions associated with the spectacular economic growth avoided a regression of average life expectancy[29].

Finally, there is a set of low-income countries, representing roughly 10% of the world's population, where both GDP and life expectancy stagnated[30]. These are the countries that are considered as "fragile states" according to the "low-income countries under stress" (LICUS) criteria for 2003–2006[31]. As much as 66% of the population in these countries is in Africa. Poor governance and extended internal conflicts are common among these countries, which all face similar hurdles: weak security, fractured societal relations, corruption, breakdown in the rule

of law, and lack of mechanisms for generating legitimate power and authority[32]. They have a huge backlog of investment needs and limited government resources to meet them. Half of them experienced negative GDP growth during the period 1995–2004 (all the others remained below the average growth of low-income countries), while their external debt was above average[33]. These countries were among those with the lowest life expectancy at birth in 1975 and have experienced minimal increases since then. The other low-income African countries share many of the characteristics and circumstances of the fragile states – in fact many of them have suffered protracted periods of conflict over the last 30 years that would have classified them as fragile states had the LICUS classification existed at that time. Their economic growth has been very limited, as has been their life-expectancy gain, not least because of the presence, in this group, of a number of southern African countries that are disproportionally confronted by the HIV/AIDS pandemic. On average, the latter have seen some economic growth since 1975, but a marked reversal in terms of life expectancy.

What has been strikingly common to fragile states and sub-Saharan African countries for much of the last three decades, and differentiates them from the others that started out with less than I$ 3000 per capita in 1975, is the combination of stagnating economic growth, political instability and lack of progress in life expectancy. They accumulate characteristics that hamper improvement of health. Education, particularly of females, develops more slowly, as does access to modern communications and knowledge-intensive work that broadens people's intellectual resources elsewhere. People are more exposed and more vulnerable to environmental and other health threats that, in today's globalized world, include lifestyle threats, such as smoking, obesity and urban violence. They lack the material security required to invest in their own health and their governments lack the necessary resources and/or commitment to public investment. They are at much greater risk of war and civil conflict than richer countries[30].

Without growth, peace is considerably more difficult and without peace, growth stagnates: on average, a civil war reduces a country's growth by around 2.3% per year for a typical duration of seven years, leaving it 15% poorer[34].

The impact of the combination of stagnation and conflicts cannot be overstated. Conflicts are a direct source of considerable excessive suffering, disease and mortality. In the Democratic Republic of the Congo, for example, the 1998–2004 conflict caused an excess mortality of 450 000 deaths per year[35]. Any strategy to close the health gaps between countries – and to correct inequalities within countries – has to give consideration to the creation of an environment of peace, stability and prosperity that allows for investment in the health sector.

A history of poor economic growth is also a history of stagnating resources for health. What

---

Box 1.2 Higher spending on health is associated with better outcomes, but with large differences between countries

In many countries, the total amount spent on health is insufficient to finance access for all to even a very limited package of essential health care[39]. This is bound to make a difference to health and survival. Figure 1.6 shows that Kenya has a health-adjusted life expectancy (HALE) of 44.4 years, the median for countries that currently spend less than I$ 100 per capita on health. This is 27 years less than Germany, the median for countries that spend more than I$ 2500 per capita. Every I$ 100 per capita spent on heath corresponds to a 1.1-year gain in HALE.

However, this masks large differences in outcomes at comparable levels of spending. There are up to five years difference in HALE between countries that spend more than I$ 2500 per capita per year on health. The spread is wider at lower expenditure levels, even within rather narrow spending bands. Inhabitants of Moldova, for example, enjoy 24 more HALE years than those of Haiti, yet they are both among the 28 countries that spend I$ 250–500 per capita on health. These gaps can even be wider if one also considers countries that are heavily affected by HIV/AIDS. Lesotho spends more on health than Jamaica, yet its people have a HALE that is 34 years shorter. In contrast, the differences in HALE between the countries with the best outcomes in each

spending band are comparatively small. Tajikistan, for example, has a HALE that is 4.3 years less than that of Sweden – less than the difference between Sweden and the United States. These differences suggest that how, for what and for whom money is spent matters considerably. Particularly in countries where the envelope for health is very small, every dollar that is allocated sub-optimally seems to make a disproportionate difference.

Figure 1.6 Countries grouped according to their total health expenditure in 2005 (international $)[38,40]

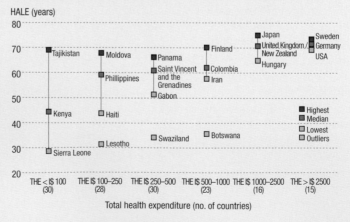

---

happened in sub-Saharan Africa during the years following Alma-Ata exemplifies this predicament. After adjusting for inflation, GDP per capita in sub-Saharan Africa fell in most years from 1980–1994[36], leaving little room to expand access to health care or transform health systems. By the early 1980s, for example, the medicines budget in the Democratic Republic of the Congo, then Zaïre, was reduced to zero and government disbursements to health districts dropped below US$ 0.1 per inhabitant; Zambia's public sector health budget was cut by two thirds; and funds available for operating expenses and salaries for the expanding government workforce dropped by up to 70% in countries such as Cameroon, Ghana, Sudan and the United Republic of Tanzania[36]. For health authorities in this part of the world, the 1980s and 1990s were a time of managing shrinking government budgets and disinvestment. For the people, this period of fiscal contraction was a time of crippling out-of-pocket payments for under-funded and inadequate health services.

In much of the world, the health sector is often massively under-funded. In 2005, 45 countries spent less than I$ 100 per capita on health, including external assistance[38]. In contrast, 16 high-income countries spent more than I$ 3000 per capita. Low-income countries generally allocate a smaller proportion of their GDP to health than high-income countries, while their GDP is smaller to start with and they have higher disease burdens.

Higher health expenditure is associated with better health outcomes, but sensitive to policy choices and context (Box 1.2): where money is scarce, the effects of errors, by omission and by commission, are amplified. Where expenditure increases rapidly, however, this offers perspectives for transforming and adapting health systems which are much more limited in a context of stagnation.

Adapting to new health challenges

A globalized, urbanized and ageing world

The world has changed over the last 30 years: few would have imagined that children in Africa would now be at far more risk of dying from traffic accidents than in either the high- or the low- and middle-income countries of the European region (Figure 1.7).

Many of the changes that affect health were already under way in 1978, but they have accelerated and will continue to do so.

Thirty years ago, some 38% of the world's population lived in cities; in 2008, it is more than 50%, 3.3 billion people. By 2030, almost 5 billion people will live in urban areas. Most of the growth will be in the smaller cities of developing countries and metropolises of unprecedented size and complexity in southern and eastern Asia[42].

Although on average health indicators in cities score better than in rural areas, the enormous social and economic stratification within urban areas results in significant health inequities[43,44,45,46]. In the high-income area of Nairobi, the under-five mortality rate is below 15 per thousand, but in the Emabakasi slum of the same city the rate is 254 per thousand[47]. These and other similar examples lead to the more general observation that within developing countries, the best local governance can help produce 75 years or more of life expectancy; with poor urban governance, life expectancy can be as low as 35 years[48]. One third of the urban population today – over one billion people – lives in slums: in places that lack durable housing, sufficient living area, access to clean water and sanitation, and secure tenure[49]. Slums are prone to fire, floods and landslides; their inhabitants are disproportionately exposed to pollution, accidents, workplace hazards and urban violence. Loss of social

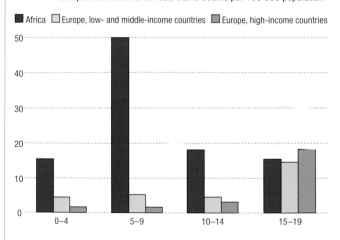

Figure 1.7 Africa's children are at more risk of dying from traffic accidents than European children: child road-traffic deaths per 100 000 population[41]

7

cohesion and globalization of unhealthy lifestyles contribute to an environment that is decidedly unfavourable for health.

These cities are where many of the world's nearly 200 million international migrants are found[50]. They constitute at least 20% of the population in 41 countries, 31% of which have less than a million inhabitants. Excluding migrants from access to care is the equivalent of denying all the inhabitants of a country similar to Brazil their rights to health. Some of the countries that have made very significant strides towards ensuring access to care for their citizens fail to offer the same rights to other residents. As migration continues to gain momentum, the entitlements of non-citizen residents and the ability of the health-care system to deal with growing linguistic and cultural diversity in equitable and effective ways are no longer marginal issues.

This mobile and urbanized world is ageing fast and will continue to do so. By 2050, the world will count 2 billion people over the age of 60, around 85% of whom will be living in today's developing countries, mostly in urban areas. Contrary to today's rich countries, low- and middle-income countries are ageing fast before having become rich, adding to the challenge.

Urbanization, ageing and globalized lifestyle changes combine to make chronic and noncommunicable diseases – including depression, diabetes, cardiovascular disease and cancers – and injuries increasingly important causes of morbidity and mortality (Figure 1.8)[51]. There is a striking shift in distribution of death and disease from younger to older ages and from infectious, perinatal and maternal causes to noncommunicable diseases. Traffic accident rates will increase; tobacco-related deaths will overtake HIV/AIDS-related deaths. Even in Africa, where the population remains younger, smoking, elevated blood pressure and cholesterol are among the top 10 risk factors in terms of overall disease burden[52]. In the last few decades, much of the lack of progress and virtually all reversals in life expectancy were associated with adult health crises, such as in the Russian Federation or southern Africa. Improved health in the future will increasingly be a question of better adult health.

Ageing has drawn attention to an issue that is of particular relevance to the organization of service delivery: the increasing frequency of multi-morbidity. In the industrialized world, as many as 25% of 65–69 year olds and 50% of 80–84 year olds are affected by two or more chronic health conditions simultaneously. In socially deprived populations, children and younger adults are also likely to be affected[53,54,55]. The frequency of multi-morbidity in low-income countries is less well described except in the context of the HIV/AIDS epidemic, malnutrition or malaria, but it is probably greatly underestimated[56,57]. As diseases of poverty are inter-related, sharing causes that

Figure 1.8 The shift towards noncommunicable diseases and accidents as causes of death*

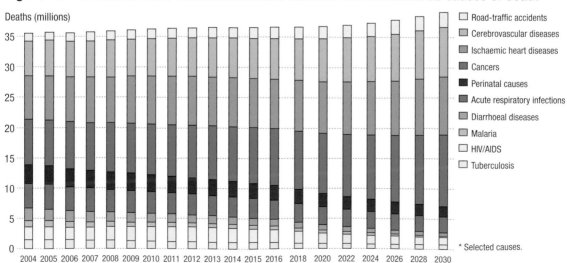

are multiple and act together to produce greater disability and ill health, multi-morbidity is probably more rather than less frequent in poor countries. Addressing co-morbidity – including mental health problems, addictions and violence – emphasizes the importance of dealing with the person as a whole. This is as important in developing countries as in the industrialized world[58].

It is insufficiently appreciated that the shift to chronic diseases or adult health has to come on top of an unfinished agenda related to communicable diseases, and maternal, newborn and child health. Efforts directed at the latter, especially in the poorest countries where coverage is still insufficient, will have to expand[12]. But all health systems, including those in the poorest countries, will also have to deal with the expanding need and demand for care for chronic and noncommunicable diseases: this is not possible without much more attention being paid to establishing a continuum of comprehensive care than is the case today. It is equally impossible without much more attention being paid to addressing the pervasive health inequalities within each country (Box 1.3).

Little anticipation and slow reactions

Over the past few decades, health authorities have shown little evidence of their ability to anticipate such changes, prepare for them or even adapt to them when they have become an everyday reality. This is worrying because the rate of change is accelerating. Globalization, urbanization and ageing will be compounded by the health effects of other global phenomena, such as climate change, the impact of which is expected to be greatest among the most vulnerable communities living in the poorest countries. Precisely how these will affect health in the coming years is more difficult to predict, but rapid changes in disease burden, growing health inequalities and disruption of social cohesion and health sector resilience are to be expected. The current food crisis has shown how unprepared health authorities often are for changes in the broader environment, even after other sectors have been sounding the alarm bell for quite some time. All too often, the accelerated pace and the global scale of the changes in the challenges to health is in contrast with the sluggish response of national health systems.

Even for well-known and documented trends, such as those resulting from the demographic and epidemiologic transitions, the level of response often remains inadequate[64]. Data from WHO's World Health Surveys, covering 18 low-income countries, show low coverage of the treatment of asthma, arthritis, angina, diabetes and depression, and of the screening for cervical and breast cancer: less than 15% in the lowest income quintile and less than 25% in the highest[65]. Public-health interventions to remove the major risk factors of disease are often neglected, even when they are particularly cost effective: they have the potential to reduce premature deaths by 47% and increase global healthy life expectancy by 9.3 years[64,66]. For example, premature tobacco-attributable deaths from ischaemic heart disease, cerebrovascular disease, chronic obstructive pulmonary disease and other diseases are projected to rise from 5.4 million in 2004 to 8.3 million in 2030, almost 10% of all deaths worldwide[67], with more than 80% in developing countries[12]. Yet, two out of every three countries are still without, or only have minimal, tobacco control policies[12].

With a few exceptions – the SARS epidemic, for example – the health sector has often been slow in dealing with new or previously underestimated health challenges. For example, awareness of the emerging health threats posed by climate change and environmental hazards dates back at least to the 1990 Earth Summit[68], but only in recent years have these begun to be translated into plans and strategies[69,70].

Health authorities have also often failed to assess, in a timely way, the significance of changes in their political environment that affect the sector's response capacity. Global and national policy environments have often taken health issues into consideration, initiating hasty and disruptive interventions, such as structural adjustment, decentralization, blueprint poverty reduction strategies, insensitive trade policies, new tax regimes, fiscal policies and the withdrawal of the state. Health authorities have a poor track record in influencing such developments, and have been ineffective in leveraging the economic weight of the health sector. Many of the critical systems issues affecting health require skills and competencies that are not found within the medical/public health establishment. The failure

Box 1.3 As information improves, the multiple dimensions of growing health inequality are becoming more apparent

In recent years, the extent of within-country disparities in vulnerability, access to care and health outcomes has been described in much greater detail (Figure 1.9)[59]. Better information shows that health inequalities tend to increase, thereby highlighting how inadequate and uneven health systems have been in responding to people's health needs. Despite the recent emphasis on poverty reduction, health systems continue to have difficulty in reaching both the rural and the urban poor, let alone addressing the multiple causes and consequences of health inequity.

Figure 1.9 Within-country inequalities in health and health care

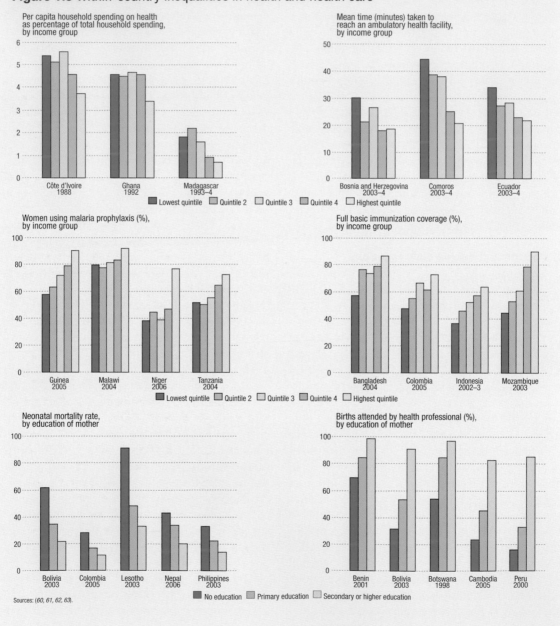

Sources: (60, 61, 62, 63).

to recognize the need for expertise from beyond traditional health disciplines has condemned the health sector to unusually high levels of systems incompetence and inefficiency which society can ill afford.

Trends that undermine the health systems' response

Without strong policies and leadership, health systems do not spontaneously gravitate towards PHC values or efficiently respond to evolving health challenges. As most health leaders know, health systems are subject to powerful forces and influences that often override rational priority setting or policy formation, thereby pulling health systems away from their intended directions[71]. Characteristic trends that shape conventional health systems today include (Figure 1.10):

- a disproportionate focus on specialist, tertiary care, often referred to as "hospital-centrism";
- fragmentation, as a result of the multiplication of programmes and projects; and
- the pervasive commercialization of health care in unregulated health systems.

With their focus on cost containment and deregulation, many of the health-sector reforms of the 1980s and 1990s have reinforced these trends. High-income countries have often been able to regulate to contain some of the adverse consequences of these trends. However, in countries where under-funding compounds

Figure 1.10 How health systems are diverted from PHC core values

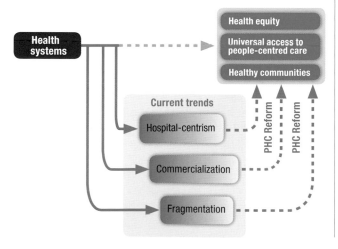

limited regulatory capacity, they have had more damaging effects.

Hospital-centrism: health systems built around hospitals and specialists

For much of the 20th century, hospitals, with their technology and sub-specialists, have gained a pivotal role in most health systems throughout the world[72,73]. Today, the disproportionate focus on hospitals and sub-specialization has become a major source of inefficiency and inequality, and one that has proved remarkably resilient. Health authorities may voice their concern more insistently than they used to, but sub-specialization continues to prevail[74]. For example, in Member countries of the Organisation of Economic Co-operation and Development (OECD), the 35% growth in the number of doctors in the last 15 years was driven by rising numbers of specialists (up by nearly 50% between 1990 and 2005 – compared with only a 20% increase in general practitioners)[75]. In Thailand, less than 20% of doctors were specialists 30 years ago; by 2003 they represented 70%[76].

The forces driving this growth include professional traditions and interests as well as the considerable economic weight of the health industry – technology and pharmaceuticals (Box 1.4). Obviously, well functioning specialized tertiary care responds to a real demand (albeit, at least in part, induced): it is necessary, at the very least, for the political credibility of the health system. However, the experience of industrialized countries has shown that a disproportionate focus on specialist, tertiary care provides poor value for money[72]. Hospital-centrism carries a considerable cost in terms of unnecessary medicalization and iatrogenesis[77], and compromises the human and social dimensions of health[73,78]. It also carries an opportunity cost: Lebanon, for example, counts more cardiac surgery units per inhabitant than Germany, but lacks programmes aimed at reducing the risk factors for cardiovascular disease[79]. Inefficient ways of dealing with health problems are thus crowding out more effective, efficient – and more equitable[80] – ways of organizing health care and improving health[81].

Since the 1980s, a majority of OECD countries has been trying to decrease reliance on hospitals,

Box 1.4 Medical equipment and pharmaceutical industries are major economic forces

Global expenditure on medical equipment and devices has grown from US$ 145 billion in 1998 to US$ 220 billion in 2006: the United States accounts for 39% of the total, the European Union for 27%, and Japan for 16%[90]. The industry employs more than 411 400 workers in the United States alone, occupying nearly one third of all the country's bioscience jobs[91]. In 2006, the United States, the European Union and Japan spent US$ 287, US$ 250 and US$ 273 per capita, respectively, on medical equipment. In the rest of the world, the average of such expenditure is in the order of US$ 6 per capita, and in sub-Saharan Africa – a market with much potential for expansion – it is US$ 2.5 per capita. The annual growth rate of the equipment market is over 10% a year[92].

The pharmaceutical industry weighs even more heavily in the global economy, with global pharmaceutical sales expected to expand to US$ 735–745 billion in 2008, with a growth rate of 6–7%[93]. Here, too, the United States is the world's largest market, accounting for around 48% of the world total: per capita expenditure on drugs was US$ 1141 in 2005, twice the level of Canada, Germany or the United Kingdom, and 10 times that of Mexico[94].

Specialized and hospital care is vital to these industries, which depend on pre-payment and risk pooling for sustainable funding of their expansion. While this market grows everywhere, there are large differences from country to country. For example, Japan and the United States have 5–8 times more magnetic resonance imaging (MRI) units per million inhabitants than Canada and the Netherlands. For computerized tomography (CT) scanners, the differences are even more pronounced: Japan had 92.6 per million in 2002, the Netherlands 5.8 in 2005[95]. These differences show that the market can be influenced, principally by using appropriate payment and reimbursement incentives and by careful consideration of the organization of regulatory control[96].

specialists and technologies, and keep costs under control. They have done this by introducing supply-side measures including reduction of hospital beds, substitution of hospitalization by home care, rationing of medical equipment, and a multitude of financial incentives and disincentives to promote micro-level efficiency. The results of these efforts have been mixed, but the evolving technology is accelerating the shift from specialized hospital to primary care. In many high-income countries (but not all), the PHC efforts of the 1980s and 1990s have been able to reach

a better balance between specialized curative care, first contact care and health promotion[81]. Over the last 30 years, this has contributed to significant improvements in health outcomes[81,82]. More recently, middle-income countries, such as Chile with its *Atención Primaria de Salud* (Primary Health Care)[83], Brazil with its family health initiative and Thailand under its universal coverage scheme[84] have shifted the balance between specialized hospital and primary care in the same way[85]. The initial results are encouraging: improvement of outcome indicators[86] combined with a marked improvement in patient satisfaction[87]. In each of these cases, the shift took place as part of a move towards universal coverage, with expanded citizen's rights to access and social protection. These processes are very similar to what occurred in Malaysia and Portugal: right to access, social protection, and a better balance between reliance on hospitals and on generalist primary care, including prevention and health promotion[6].

Industrialized countries are, 50 years later, trying to reduce their reliance on hospitals, having realized the opportunity cost of hospital-centrism in terms of effectiveness and equity. Yet, many low- and middle-income countries are creating the same distortions. The pressure from consumer demand, the medical professions and the medico-industrial complex[88] is such that private *and* public health resources flow disproportionately towards specialized hospital care at the expense of investment in primary care. National health authorities have often lacked the financial and political clout to curb this trend and achieve a better balance. Donors have also used their influence more towards setting up disease control programmes than towards reforms that would make primary care the hub of the health system[89].

Fragmentation: health systems built around priority programmes

While urban health by and large revolves around hospitals, the rural poor are increasingly confronted with the progressive fragmentation of their health services, as "selective" or "vertical" approaches focus on individual disease control programmes and projects. Originally considered as an interim strategy to achieve equitable health outcomes, they sprang from a concern for the slow expansion of access to health care in a context of persistent severe excess mortality and morbidity for which cost-effective interventions exist[97]. A focus on programmes and projects is particularly attractive to an international community concerned with getting a visible return on investment. It is well adapted to command-and-control management: a way of working that also appeals to traditional ministries of health. With little tradition of collaboration with other stakeholders and participation of the public, and with poor capacity for regulation, programmatic approaches have been a natural channel for developing governmental action in severely resource-constrained and donor-dependent countries. They have had the merit of focusing on health care in severely resource-constrained circumstances, with welcome attention to reaching the poorest and those most deprived of services.

Many have hoped that single-disease control initiatives would maximize return on investment and somehow strengthen health systems as interventions were delivered to large numbers of people, or would be the entry point to start building health systems where none existed. Often the opposite has proved true. The limited sustainability of a narrow focus on disease control, and the distortions it causes in weak and under-funded health systems have been criticized extensively in recent years[98]. Short-term advances have been short-lived and have fragmented health services to a degree that is now of major concern to health authorities. With parallel chains of command and funding mechanisms, duplicated supervision and training schemes, and multiplied transaction costs, they have led to situations where programmes compete for scarce resources, staff and donor attention, while the structural problems of health systems – funding, payment and human resources – are hardly addressed. The discrepancy in salaries between regular public sector jobs and better-funded programmes and projects has exacerbated the human resource crisis in fragile health systems. In Ethiopia, contract staff hired to help implement programmes were paid three times more than regular government employees[99], while in Malawi, a hospital saw 88 nurses leave for better paid nongovernmental organization (NGO) programmes in an 18 month period[100].

Eventually, service delivery ends up dealing only with the diseases for which a (funded) programme exists – overlooking people who have the misfortune not to fit in with current programme priorities. It is difficult to maintain the people's trust if they are considered as mere programme targets. services then lack social sustainability. This is not just a problem for the population. It puts health workers in the unenviable position of having to turn down people with "the wrong kind of problem" – something that fits ill with the self-image of professionalism and caring many cherish. Health authorities may at first be seduced by the straightforwardness of programme funding and management, yet once programmes multiply and fragmentation becomes unmanageable and unsustainable, the merits of more integrated approaches are much more evident. The re-integration of programmes once they have been well established is no easy task.

Health systems left to drift towards unregulated commercialization

In many, if not most low- and middle-income countries, under-resourcing and fragmentation of health services has accelerated the development of commercialized health care, defined here as the unregulated fee-for-service sale of health care, regardless of whether or not it is supplied by public, private or NGO providers.

Commercialization of health care has reached previously unheard of proportions in countries that, by choice or due to a lack of capacity, fail to regulate the health sector. Originally limited to an urban phenomenon, small-scale unregulated fee-for-service health care offered by a multitude of different independent providers now dominates the health-care landscape from sub-Saharan Africa to the transitional economies in Asia or Europe.

Commercialization often cuts across the public-private divide[101]. Health-care delivery in many governmental and even in traditionally not-for-profit NGO facilities has been de facto commercialized, as informal payment systems and cost-recovery systems have shifted the cost of services to users in an attempt to compensate for the chronic under-funding of the public health sector and the fiscal stringency of structural adjustment[102,103]. In these same countries, moonlighting civil servants make up a considerable part of the unregulated commercial sector[104], while others resort to under-the-counter payments[105,106,107]. The public-private debate of the last decades has, thus, largely missed the point: for the people, the real issue is not whether their health-care provider is a public employee or a private entrepreneur, nor whether health facilities are publicly or privately owned. Rather, it is whether or not health services are reduced to a commodity that can be bought and sold on a fee-for-service basis without regulation or consumer protection[108].

Commercialization has consequences for quality as well as for access to care. The reasons are straightforward: the provider has the knowledge; the patient has little or none. The provider has an interest in selling what is most profitable, but not necessarily what is best for the patient. Without effective systems of checks and balances, the results can be read in consumer organization reports or newspaper articles that express outrage at the breach of the implicit contract of trust between caregiver and client[109]. Those who cannot afford care are excluded; those who can may not get the care they need, often get care they do not need, and invariably pay too much.

Unregulated commercialized health systems are highly inefficient and costly[110]: they exacerbate inequality[111], and they provide poor quality and, at times, dangerous care that is bad for health (in the Democratic Republic of the Congo, for example, "*la chirurgie safari*" (safari surgery) refers to a common practice of health workers moonlighting by performing appendectomies or other surgical interventions at the patients' homes, often for crippling fees).

Thus, commercialization of health care is an important contributor to the erosion of trust in health services and in the ability of health authorities to protect the public[111]. This is what makes it a matter of concern for politicians and, much more than was the case 30 years ago, one of the main reasons for increasing support for reforms that would bring health systems more in line not only with current health challenges, but also with people's expectations.

Changing values and rising expectations

The reason why health systems are organized around hospitals or are commercialized is largely because they are supply-driven and also correspond to demand: genuine as well as supply-induced. Health systems are also a reflection of a globalizing consumer culture. Yet, at the same time, there are indications that people are aware that such health systems do not provide an adequate response to need and demand, and that they are driven by interests and goals that are disconnected from people's expectations. As societies modernize and become more affluent and knowledgeable, what people consider to be desirable ways of living as individuals and as members of societies, i.e. what people value, changes[112]. People tend to regard health services more as a commodity today, but they also have other, rising expectations regarding health and health care. People care more about health as an integral part of how they and their families go about their everyday lives than is commonly thought (Box 1.5)[113]. They expect their families and communities to be protected from risks and dangers to health. They want health care that deals with people as individuals with rights and not as mere targets for programmes or beneficiaries of charity. They are willing to respect health professionals but want to be respected in turn, in a climate of mutual trust[114].

People also have expectations about the way their society deals with health and health care. They aspire to greater health equity and solidarity and are increasingly intolerant of social exclusion – even if individually they may be reluctant to act on these values[115]. They expect health authorities – whether in government or other bodies – to do more to protect their right to health. The social values surveys that have been conducted since the 1980s show increasing convergence in this regard between the values of developing countries and of more affluent societies, where protection of health and access to care is often taken for granted[112,115,116]. Increasing prosperity, access to knowledge and social connectivity are associated with rising expectations. People want to have more say about what happens in their workplace, in the communities in which they live and also in important government decisions that

Box 1.5 Health is among the top personal concerns

When people are asked to name the most important problems that they and their families are currently facing, financial worries often come out on top, with health a close second[118]. In one country out of two, personal illness, health-care costs, poor quality care or other health issues are the top personal concerns of over one third of the population surveyed (Figure 1.11). It is, therefore, not surprising that a breakdown of the health-care system – or even the hint of a breakdown – can lead to popular discontent that threatens the ambitions of the politicians seen to be responsible[119].

Figure 1.11 Percentage of the population citing health as their main concern before other issues, such as financial problems, housing or crime[118]

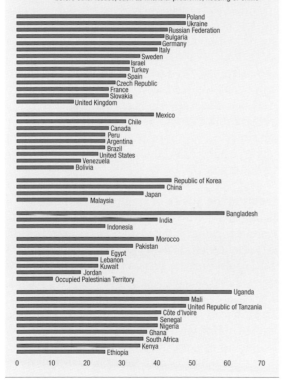

affect their lives[117]. The desire for better care and protection of health, for less health inequity and for participation in decisions that affect health is more widespread and more intense now than it was 30 years ago. Therefore, much more is expected of health authorities today.

Health equity

Equity, whether in health, wealth or power is rarely, if ever, fully achieved. Some societies are more egalitarian than others, but on the whole the world is "unequal". Value surveys, however, clearly demonstrate that people care about these inequalities – considering a substantial proportion to be unfair "inequities" that can and should be avoided. Data going back to the early 1980s show that people increasingly disagree with the way in which income is distributed and believe that a "just society" should work to correct these imbalances[120,121,122,123]. This gives policy-makers less leeway to ignore the social dimensions of their policies than they might have had previously[120,124].

People are often unaware of the full scope of health inequalities. Most Swedish citizens, for example, were probably unaware that the difference in life expectancy between 20-year-old men from the highest and lowest socioeconomic groups was 3.97 years in 1997: a gap that had widened by 88% compared to 1980[125]. However, while people's knowledge on these topics may be partial, research shows that people regard social gradients in health as profoundly unjust[126]. Intolerance to inequality in health and to the exclusion of population groups from health benefits and social protection mirrors or exceeds intolerance to inequality in income. In most societies, there is wide consensus that everybody should be able to take care of their health and to receive treatment when ill or injured – without being bankrupted and pushed into poverty[127].

As societies become wealthier, popular support for equitable access to health care and social protection to meet basic health and social needs gains stronger ground. Social surveys show that, in the European region, 93% of the populations support comprehensive health coverage[117]. In the United States, long reputed for its reluctance to adopt a national health insurance system, more than 80% of the population is in favour of it[115], while basic care for all continues to be a widely distributed, intensely held, social goal[128]. The attitudes in lower income countries are less well known, but extrapolating from their views on income inequality, it is reasonable to assume that increasing prosperity is coupled with rising concern for health equity – even if consensus about how this should be achieved may be as contentious as in richer countries.

Care that puts people first

People obviously want effective health care when they are sick or injured. They want it to come from providers with the integrity to act in their best interests, equitably and honestly, with knowledge and competence. The demand for competence is not trivial: it fuels the health economy with steadily increased demand for professional care (doctors, nurses and other non-physician clinicians who play an increasing role in both industrialized and developing countries)[129]. For example, throughout the world, women are switching from the use of traditional birth attendants to midwives, doctors and obstetricians (Figure 1.12)[130].

The PHC movement has underestimated the speed with which the transition in demand from traditional caregivers to professional care would bypass initial attempts to rapidly expand access to health care by relying on non-professional "community health workers", with their added value of cultural competence. Where strategies for extending PHC coverage proposed lay workers as an alternative rather than as a complement to professionals, the care provided has often been perceived to be poor[131]. This has pushed people towards commercial care, which they, rightly or wrongly, perceived to be more competent, while attention was diverted from the challenge of more effectively incorporating professionals under the umbrella of PHC.

Proponents of PHC were right about the importance of cultural and relational competence, which was to be the key comparative advantage of community health workers. Citizens in the developing world, like those in rich countries, are not looking for technical competence alone: they also want health-care providers to be understanding, respectful and trustworthy[132]. They want health care to be organized around their needs, respectful of their beliefs and sensitive to their particular situation in life. They do not want to be taken advantage of by unscrupulous providers, nor do they want to be considered mere targets for disease control programmes (they may never have liked that, but they are now certainly becoming more vocal about it). In poor and rich countries, people want more from health care than interventions. Increasingly, there is recognition that the resolution of health problems should take into account the socio-cultural context of the families and communities where they occur[133].

Much public and private health care today is organized around what providers consider to be effective and convenient, often with little attention to or understanding of what is important for their clients[134]. Things do not have to be that way. As experience – particularly from industrialized countries – has shown, health services can be made more people-centred. This makes them more effective and also provides a more rewarding working environment[135]. Regrettably, developing countries have often put less emphasis on making services more people-centred, as if this were less relevant in resource-constrained circumstances. However, neglecting people's needs and expectations is a recipe for disconnecting health services from the communities they serve. People-centredness is not a luxury, it is a necessity, also for services catering to the poor. Only people-centred services will minimize social exclusion and avoid leaving people at the mercy of unregulated commercialized health care, where the illusion of a more responsive environment carries a hefty price in terms of financial expense and iatrogenesis.

Securing the health of communities

People do not think about health only in terms of sickness or injury, but also in terms of what they perceive as endangering their health and that of their community[118]. Whereas cultural and political explanations for health hazards vary widely, there is a general and growing tendency to hold the authorities responsible for offering protection against, or rapidly responding to such dangers[136]. This is an essential part of the social contract that gives legitimacy to the state. Politicians in rich as well as poor countries increasingly ignore their duty to protect people from health hazards at their peril: witness the political fall-out of the poor management of the hurricane Katrina disaster in the United States in 2005, or of the 2008 garbage disposal crisis in Naples, Italy.

Access to information about health hazards in our globalizing world is increasing. Knowledge is spreading beyond the community of health professionals and scientific experts. Concerns about health hazards are no longer limited to the traditional public health agenda of improving

Figure 1.12 The professionalization of birthing care: percentage of births assisted by professional and other carers in selected areas, 2000 and 2005 with projections to 2015[a]

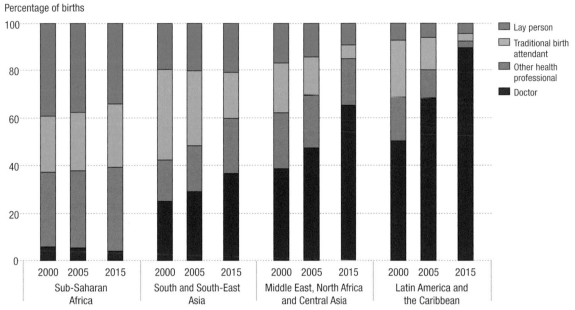

[a] Source: Pooled data from 88 DHS surveys 1995–2006, linear projection to 2015.

the quality of drinking water and sanitation to prevent and control infectious diseases. In the wake of the 1986 Ottawa Charter for Health Promotion[137], a much wider array of issues constitute the health promotion agenda, including food safety and environmental hazards as well as collective lifestyles, and the social environment that affects health and quality of life[138]. In recent years, it has been complemented by growing concerns for a health hazard that used to enjoy little visibility, but is increasingly the object of media coverage: the risks to the safety of patients[139].

Reliable, responsive health authorities

During the 20th century, health has progressively been incorporated as a public good guaranteed by government entitlement. There may be disagreement as to how broadly to define the welfare state and the collective goods that go with it[140,141], but, in modernizing states, the social and political responsibility entrusted to health authorities – not just ministries of health, but also local governmental structures, professional organizations and civil society organizations with a quasi-governmental role – is expanding.

Circumstances or short-term political expediency may at times tempt governments to withdraw from their social responsibilities for financing and regulating the health sector, or from service delivery and essential public health functions. Predictably, this creates more problems than it solves. Whether by choice or because of external pressure, the withdrawal of the state that occurred in the 1980s and 1990s in China and the former Soviet Union, as well as in a considerable number of low-income countries, has had visible and worrisome consequences for health and for the functioning of health services. Significantly, it has created social tensions that affected the legitimacy of political leadership[119].

In many parts of the world, there is considerable skepticism about the way and the extent to which health authorities assume their responsibilities for health. Surveys show a trend of diminishing trust in public institutions as guarantors of the equity, honesty and integrity of the health sector[123,142,143]. Nevertheless, on the whole, people expect their health authorities to work for the common good, to do this well and with foresight[144]. There is a multiplication of scoring cards, rankings and other league tables of public action used either at the national or global level[141], while consumer organizations are addressing health sector problems[111], and national and global civil society watchdog organizations are emerging[146,147,148,149]. These recent trends attest to prevailing doubts about how well health authorities are able to provide stewardship for the health system, as well as to the rising expectations for them to do even better.

Participation

At the same time, however, surveys show that, as societies modernize, people increasingly want to "have a say" in "important decisions that affect their lives"[123,112], which would include issues such as resource allocation and the organization and regulation of care. Experience from countries as diverse as Chile, Sweden and Thailand shows, however, that people are more concerned with having guarantees for fair and transparent processes than with the actual technicalities of priority setting[150,151]. In other words, an optimum response to aspirations for a bigger say in health policy matters would be evidence of a structured and functional system of checks and balances. This would include relevant stakeholders and would guarantee that the policy agenda could not be hijacked by particular interest groups[152].

PHC reforms: driven by demand

The core values articulated by the PHC movement three decades ago are, thus, more powerfully present in many settings now than at the time of Alma-Ata. They are not just there in the form of moral convictions espoused by an intellectual vanguard. Increasingly, they exist as concrete social expectations felt and asserted by broad groups of ordinary citizens within modernizing societies. Thirty years ago, the values of equity, people-centredness, community participation and self-determination embraced by the PHC movement were considered radical by many. Today, these values have become widely shared social expectations for health that increasingly pervade many of the world's societies – though the language people use to express these expectations may differ from that of Alma-Ata.

This evolution from formal ethical principles to generalized social expectations fundamentally alters the political dynamics around health systems change. It opens fresh opportunities for generating social and political momentum to move health systems in the directions people want them to go, and that are summarized in Figure 1.13. It moves the debate from a purely technical discussion on the relative efficiency of various ways of "treating" health problems to include political considerations on the social goals that define the direction in which to steer health systems. The subsequent chapters outline a set of reforms aimed at aligning specialist-based, fragmented and commercialized health systems with these rising social expectations. These PHC reforms aim to channel society's resources towards more equity and an end to exclusion; towards health services that revolve around people's needs and expectations; and towards public policies that secure the health of communities. Across these reforms is the imperative of engaging citizens and other stakeholders: recognizing that vested interests that tend to pull health systems in different directions raises the premium on leadership and vision and on sustained learning to do better.

Figure 1.13 The social values that drive PHC and the corresponding sets of reforms

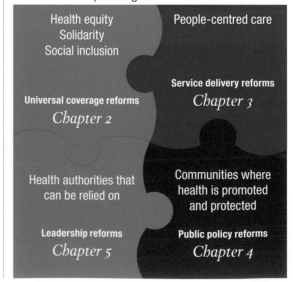

Health equity
Solidarity
Social inclusion

People-centred care

Universal coverage reforms
Chapter 2

Service delivery reforms
Chapter 3

Health authorities that can be relied on

Communities where health is promoted and protected

Leadership reforms
Chapter 5

Public policy reforms
Chapter 4

References

1. Smith R. Oman: leaping across the centuries. *British Medical Journal*, 1988, 297:540–544.
2. *Sultanate of Oman: second primary health care review mission*. Geneva, World Health Organization, 2006.
3. *Primary health care performance*. Muscat, Sultanate of Oman. Directorate General of Health Affairs, Department of Primary Health Care, 2006.
4. Infante A. *The post military government reforms to the Chilean health system. A case study commissioned by the Health Systems Knowledge Network. Paper presented in the Health Services Knowledge Network Meeting, London, October 2006*. Geneva, World Health Organization, Commission on the Social Determinants of Health, 2007.
5. Pathmanathan I, Dhairiam S. Malaysia: moving from infectious to chronic diseases. In: Tarimo E, ed. *Achieving health for all by the year 2000: midway reports of country experiences*. Geneva, World Health Organization, 1990.
6. Biscaia A et al. *Cuidados de saúde primários em Portugal: reformar para novos sucessos*. Lisbon, Padrões Culturais Editora, 2006.
7. Pongsupap Y. *Introducing a human dimension to Thai health care: the case for family practice*. Brussels, Vrije Universiteit Brussel Press, 2007.
8. Barros P, Simões J. *Portugal: health system review*. Geneva, World Health Organization Regional Office for Europe on behalf of the European Observatory of Health Systems and Policies, 2007 (Health Systems in Transition No. 9; http://www.euro.who.int/Document/E90670.pdf, accessed 1 July 2008).
9. Bentes M, Dias CM, Sakellarides C, Bankauskaite V. *Health care systems in transition: Portugal*. Copenhagen, World Health Organization Regional Office for Europe on behalf of the European Observatory on Health Systems and Policies, 2004 (Health Care Systems in Transition No. 1; http://www.euro.who.int/document/e82937.pdf, accessed 1 June 2000).
10. Ferrinho P, Bugalho M, Miguel JP. eds. *For better health in Europe, Vol. 1*. Lisbon, Fundação Merck Sharp & Dohme, 2004.
11. Biscaia A et al. *Cuidados de saúde primários portugueses e a mortalidade vulnerável às intervenções dos serviços de saúde – o caso português* [Portuguese primary health care and health services intervention in mortality amenable to health service intervention. Geneva, World Health Organization 2008 (unpublished background paper for the *World Health Report 2008 – Primary health care: now more than ever*, Geneva, World Health Organization, 2008).
12. *World Health Statistics 2008*. Geneva, World Health Organization, 2008.
13. Murray CJL et al. Can we achieve Millennium Development Goal 4? New analysis of country trends and forecasts of under-5 mortality to 2015. *Lancet* 2007, 370:1040–1054.
14. *The Millennium Development Goals report 2007*. New York, United Nations, 2007 (http://www.un.org/millenniumgoals/pdf/mdg2007.pdf, accessed 1 July 2008).
15. *Levels and trends of contraceptive use as assessed in 2002*. New York, United Nations, Department of Economic and Social Affairs, Population Division, 2004 (Sales No. E.04.XIII.9).
16. *World contraceptive use 2007, wall chart*. New York, United Nations, Department of Economic and Social Affairs, Population Division, 2008 (Sales No. E.08.XIII.6).
17. Sedgh G et al. Induced abortion: estimated rates and trends worldwide. *Lancet, 2007,* 370:1338–1345.
18. Koblinsky M et al. Going to scale with professional skilled care. *Lancet*, 2006, 368:1377–1386.
19. Goesling B, Ferebaugh G. The trend in international health inequality. *Population and Development Review*, 2004, 30:131–146.
20. Preston S. The changing relation between mortality and level of economic development. *Population Studies*, 1975, 29:231–248.
21. *The state of the world's children 2008*. Paris, United Nations Children's Fund, 2008.
22. Cutler DM, Deaton A, Lleras-Muney A. *The determinants of mortality*. Cambridge, MA, National Bureau of Economic Research, 2006 (NBER Working Paper No. 11963).
23. Deaton A. *Global patterns of income and health: facts, interpretations, and policies, WIDER Annual Lecture, Helsinki, September 29th, 2006*. Princeton NJ, Princeton University Press, 2006.
24. Field M, Shkolnikov V. Russia: socioeconomic dimensions of the gender gap in mortality. In: Evans et al. *Challenging inequities in health: from ethics to action*. New York, Oxford University Press 2001.
25. WHO mortality database: tables [online database]. Geneva, World Health Organization, 2007 (http://www.who.int/healthinfo/morttables/en/index.html, accessed 1 July 2008).
26. Suhrcke M, Rocco L, McKee M. *Health: a vital investment for economic development in eastern Europe and central Asia*. European Observatory on Health Systems and Policies, 2008 (http://www.euro.who.int/observatory/Publications/20070618_1, accessed 1 July 2008).
27. Banister J, Zhang X. China, economic development and mortality decline. *World Development*, 2005, 33:21–41.
28. Banister J, Hill K. Mortality in China, 1964-2000. *Population studies*, 2004, 58:55–75.
29. Gu D et al. *Decomposing changes in life expectancy at birth by age, sex and residence from 1929 to 2000 in China. Paper present at the American Population Association 2007 annual meeting, New York, 29-31 March 2007* (unpublished).
30. Milanovic B. *Why did the poorest countries fail to catch up?* Washington DC, Carnegie Endowment for International Peace, 2005 (Carnegie Paper No. 62).
31. Carvalho S. *Engaging with fragile states: an IEG review of World Bank support to low-income countries under stress. Appendix B: LICUS, fiscal 2003-06*. Washington DC, The World Bank, 2006 (http://www.worldbank.org/ieg/licus/docs/appendix_b.pdf, accessed 1 July 2008).
32. Carvalho S. *Engaging with fragile states: an IEG review of World Bank support to low-income countries under stress. Chapter 3: Operational utility of the LICUS identification, classification, and aid-allocation system*. Washington DC, The World Bank, 2006 (http://www.worldbank.org/ieg/licus/docs/licus_chap3.pdf, accessed 1 July 2008).
33. Ikpe, E. Challenging the discourse on fragile states. *Conflict, Security and Development*, 2007, 77:84–124.
34. Collier P. *The bottom billion: why the poorest countries are failing and what can be done about it*. New York, Oxford University Press, 2007.
35. Coghlan B et al. Mortality in the Democratic Republic of Congo: a nationwide survey. *Lancet*, 2006, 367:44–51.
36. *World development indicators 2007*. Washington DC, The World Bank, 2007 (http://go.worldbank.org/3JU2HA60D0, accessed 1 July 2008).
37. Van Lerberghe W, De Brouwere V. État de sante et santé de l'État en Afrique subsaharienne [State of health and health of the state in sub-Saharan Africa], *Afrique Contemporaine*, 2000, 135:175–190.
38. National health accounts country information for 2002–2005. Geneva, World Health Organization, 2008 (http://www.who.int/nha/country/en, accessed 2 July 2008).
39. Xu K et al. Protecting households from catastrophic health expenditures, *Health Affairs*, 2007, 26:972–983.
40. *The World Health Report 2004 – Changing history: overview. Annex table 4: healthy life expectancy in WHO Member States, estimates for 2002*. Geneva, World Health Organization, 2004 (http://www.who.int/whr/2004/annex/topic/en/annex_4_en.pdf, accessed 2 July 2008).
41. *WHO global burden of disease estimates: 2004 update*. Geneva, World Health Organization, 2008 (http://www.who.int/healthinfo/bodestimates/en/index.html, accessed 2 July 2008).
42. *State of world population 2007. Unleashing the potential of urban growth*. New York, United Nations Population Fund, 2007.
43. Vlahov D et al. Urban as a determinant of health. *Journal of Urban Health*, 2007, 84(Suppl. 1):16–26.
44. Montgomery M, Hewett, PC. *Urban poverty and health in developing countries: household and neighborhood effects demography*. New York, The Population Council, 2004 (Policy Research Division Working paper No. 184; http://www.popcouncil.org/pdfs/wp/184.pdf, accessed 1 July 2008).
45. Satterthwaite D. *Coping with rapid urban growth*. London, Royal Institution of Chartered Surveyors, 2002 (RICS Leading Edge Series; POPLINE Document No. 180006).
46. Garenne M, Gakusi E. Health transitions in sub-Saharan Africa: overview of mortality trends in children under 5 years old (1950–2000). *Bulletin of the World Health Organization*, 2006, 84:470–478.
47. *Population and health dynamics in Nairobi's informal settlements*. Nairobi, African Population and Health Research Center Inc., 2002.
48. *Report of the knowledge network on urban settlement*. Geneva, World Health Organization, Commission on Social Determinants of Health, 2008.
49. *State of world population 2007. Unleashing the potential of urban growth*. New York, United Nations Population Fund, 2007.
50. *International Migration Report 2006*. 2006. New York, United Nations, Department of Economic and Social Affairs, 2006.
51. Abegunde D et al. The burden and costs of chronic diseases in low-income and middle-income countries. *Lancet*, 2007, 370:1929–1938.
52. *The World Health Report 2002 – Reducing risks, promoting healthy life*. Geneva, World Health Organization, 2002.
53. Amaducci L, Scarlato G, Candalese L. *Italian longitudinal study on ageing. ILSA resource data book*. Rome, Consiglio Nazionale per le Ricerche, 1996.

54. Marengoni A. *Prevalence and impact of chronic diseases and multimorbidity in the ageing population: a clinical and epidemiological approach*. Stockholm, Karolinska Institutet, 2008.

55. McWhinney I. The essence of general practice. In: Lakhani M, ed. *A celebration of general practice*. London, Royal College of General Practitioners, 2003.

56. Kazembe LN, Namangale JJ. A Bayesian multinomial model to analyse spatial patterns of childhood co-morbidity in Malawi. *European Journal of Epidemiology*, 2007, 22:545–556.

57. Gwer S, Newton CR, Berkley JA. Over-diagnosis and co-morbidity of severe malaria in African children: a guide for clinicians. *American Journal of Tropical Medicine and Hygiene*. 2007 77(Suppl. 6):6–13.

58. Starfield B et al. Comorbidity: implications for the importance of primary care in 'case' management. *Annals of Family Medicine*, 2003, 1:814.

59. Gwatkin D et al. *Socio-economic differences in health nutrition and population*. Washington DC, The World Bank, 2000 (Health Nutrition and Population Discussion Paper).

60. Castro-Leal F et al. Public spending on health care in Africa: do the poor benefit? *Bulletin of the World Health Organization*, 2000, 78:66–74.

61. World Health Surveys. Geneva, World Health Organization, 2008.

62. STATcompiler [online database]. Calverton MD, Demographic Health Surveys, 2008 (http://www.statcompiler.com/, accessed 22 July 2008).

63. Davidson R et al. *Country report on HNP and poverty – socio-economic differences in health, nutrition, and population within developing countries: an overview. Produced by the World Bank in collaboration with the government of the Netherlands and the Swedish International Development Cooperation Agency*. Washington DC, The World Bank, 2007.

64. Strong K et al. Preventing chronic diseases: how many lives can we save? *Lancet*, 366:1578–1582.

65. *World health survey: internal calculations*. Geneva, World Health Organization, 2008 (unpublished).

66. Ezzati M et al. Comparative risk assessment collaborating group. Estimates of global and regional potential health gains from reducing multiple major risk factors. *Lancet,* 2003, 362:271–280.

67. *WHO report on the global tobacco epidemic, 2008: the MPOWER package*. Geneva, World Health Organization, 2008.

68. Bettcher DW, Sapirie S, Goon EH. Essential public health functions: results of the international Delphi study, *World Health Stat Q*, 1998, 51:44–54.

69. *The World Health Report 2007 – A safer future, global public health security in the 21st century*. Geneva, World Health Organization, 2007.

70. Rockenschaub G, Pukkila J, Profili M. *Towards health security. A discussion paper on recent health crises in the WHO European Region*. Copenhagen, World Health Organization Regional Office for Europe, 2007.

71. Moran M. *Governing the health care state. A comparative study of the United Kingdom, the United States and Germany*. Manchester, Manchester University Press, 1999.

72. Starfield B. *Primary care. Balancing health needs, services and technology*. New York, Oxford University Press, 1998.

73. Pongsupap Y. *Introducing a human dimension to Thai health care: the case for family practice*. Brussels, Vrije Universiteit Brussel Press, 2007.

74. Brotherton SE, Rockey PH, Etzel SI. US graduate medical education, 2004-2005: trends in primary care specialties. *Journal of the American Medical Association*, 2005, 294:1075–1082.

75. OECD Health Data 2007. SourceOECD [online database]. Paris, Organisation for Economic Co-operation and Development, 18 July 2007 (http://www.oecd.org/doc ument/10/0,3343,en_2649_37407_38976778_1_1_1_37407,00.html, accessed 1 July 2008).

76. Jindawatthana A, Jongudomsul P. Human resources for health and universal health care coverage. Thailand's experience. *Journal for Human Resources for Health* (forthcoming).

77. The Research Priority Setting Working Group of the WHO World Alliance for Patient Safety. *Summary of the evidence on patient safety. Implications for research*. Geneva, World Health Organization, 2008.

78. Liamputtong P. Giving birth in the hospital: childbirth experiences of Thai women in northern Thailand. *Health Care for Women International*, 2004, 25:454–480.

79. Ammar W. *Health system and reform in Lebanon*. Beirut, World Health Organization Regional Office for the Eastern Mediterranean, 2003.

80. Whitehead M, Dahlgren G. *Concepts and principles for tackling social inequities in health: Levelling up part 1*. Copenhagen, World Health Organization Regional Office for Europe, 2006. (Studies on Social and Economic Determinants of Population Health No. 2; http://www.euro.who.int/document/e89383.pdf, accessed 15 July 2008).

81. Starfield B, Shi L. Policy relevant determinants of health: an international perspective. *Health Policy*, 2002, 60:201–218.

82. Schoen C et al. 2006 US health system performance: a national scorecard. *Health Affairs*, 20 September *2006* (Web Exclusive, w457–w475).

83. Gobierno de Chile. Ministerio de Salud. *Orientaciones para la programación en red*. Santiago, Subsecretaria de Redes Asistenciales, Division de Gestion de Red Asistencial, 2006.

84. Suraratdecha C, Saithanu S, Tangcharoensathien V. Is universal coverage a solution for disparities in health care? Findings from three low-income provinces of Thailand. *Health Policy*, 73:272–284.

85. Tangcharoensathien V et al. Knowledge-based changes to the Thai health system. *Bulletin of the World Health Organization*, 2004, 82:750–756.

86. Macinko J et al. Going to scale with community-based primary care: an analysis of the family health program and infant mortality in Brazil, 1999–2004. *Social Science & Medicine*, 2007, 65:2070–2080.

87. Pongsupap Y, Boonyapaisarnchoaroen T, Van Lerberghe W. The perception of patients using primary care units in comparison with conventional public hospital outpatient departments and "prime mover family practices": an exit survey. *Journal of Health Science*, 2005, 14:475–483.

88. Relman AS. The new medical-industrial complex. *New England Journal of Medicine*, 1980, 303:963–970.

89. *Aid effectiveness and health. Making health systems work*. Geneva, World Health Organization, 2007 (Working Paper 9; WHO/HSS/healthsystems/2007.2).

90. *Lifestyle and health*. EurActiv, 2006 (http://www.euractiv.com/en/health/medical-devices/article-117519, accessed 1 July2008).

91. Medical Device Statistics, *PharmaMedDevice's Bulletin*, 2006 (http://www.pharmameddevice.com/App/homepage.cfm?appname=100485&linkid=23294&mo duleid=3162#Medical_Device, accessed 1 July 2008).

92. *Medical technology industry at a glance*. Washington DC, Advanced Medical Technology Association, 2004 (http://www.advamed.org/NR/rdonlyres/0A261055-827C-4CC6-80B6-CC2D8FA04A33/0/ChartbookSept2004.pdf, accessed 15 July 2008).

93. Press room: IMS health predicts 5 to 6 percent growth for global pharmaceutical market in 2008, according to annual forecast. *IMS Intelligence Applied*, 1 November 2007 (http://www.imshealth.com/ims/portal/front/articleC/0,2777,6599_3665_82713022,00.html, accessed 1 July 2008).

94. Danzon PM, Furukawa MF. International prices and availability of pharmaceuticals in 2005. *Health Affairs*, 2005, 27:221–233.

95. *Health at a glance 2007: OECD indicators*. Paris, Organisation for Economic Co-operation and Development, 2007.

96. Moran M. *Governing the health care state. A comparative study of the United Kingdom, the United States and Germany*. Manchester, Manchester University Press, 1999.

97. Walsh JA, Warren KS. Selective primary health care: an interim strategy for disease control in developing countries. *New England Journal of Medicine*, 1979, 301:967–974.

98. Buse K, Harmer AM. Seven habits of highly effective global public–private health partnerships: Practice and potential, *Social Science & Medicine*, 2007, 64:259–271.

99. Stillman K, Bennet S. *System wide effects of the Global Fund interim findings from three country studies*. Washington DC, United States Agency for Aid and Development, 2005.

100. Malawi Ministry of Health and The World Bank. *Human resources and financing in the health sector in Malawi*. Washington DC, World Bank, 2004.

101. Giusti D, Criel B, de Béthune X. Viewpoint: public versus private health care delivery: beyond slogans. *Health Policy and Planning*, 1997, 12:193–198.

102. Périn I, Attaran A. Trading ideology for dialogue: an opportunity to fix international aid for health. *Lancet*, 2003, 362:1216–1219.

103. Creese AL. User charges for health care: a review of recent experience. Geneva, World Health Organization, 1990 (Strengthening Health Systems Paper No. 1).

104. Macq J et al. Managing health services in developing countries: between the ethics of the civil servant and the need for moonlighting. *Human Resources for Health Development Journal*, 2001, 5:17–24.

105. Delcheva E, Balabanova D, McKee M. Under-the-counter payments for health care: evidence from Bulgaria. *Health Policy*, 1997, 42:89–100.

106. João Schwalbach et al. Good Samaritan or exploiter of illness? Coping strategies of Mozambican health care providers. In: Ferrinho P, Van Lerberghe W. eds. *Providing health care under adverse conditions. Health personnel performance and individual coping strategies*. Antwerp, ITGPress, 2000.

107. Ferrinho P et al. Pilfering for survival: how health workers use access to drugs as a coping strategy. *Human Resources for Health*, 2004, 2:4.

108. McIntyre D et al. Commercialisation and extreme inequality in health: the policy challenges in South Africa. *Journal of International Development*, 2006, 18:435–446.

109. Sakboon M et al. Case studies in litigation between patients and doctors. Bangkok, The Foundation of Consumer Protection, 1999.

110. Ammar, W. *Health system and reform in Lebanon.* Beirut, World Health Organization Regional Office for the Eastern Mediterranean, 2003.

111. Macintosh M. *Planning and market regulation: strengths, weaknesses and interactions in the provision of less inequitable and better quality health care.* Geneva, World Health Organization, Health Systems Knowledge Network, Commission on the Social Determinants of Health, 2007.

112. Inglehart R, Welzel C. *Modernization, cultural change and democracy: the human development sequence.* Cambridge, Cambridge University Press, 2005.

113. Kickbush I. Innovation in health policy: responding to the health society. *Gaceta Sanitaria,* 2007, 21:338–342.

114. Anand S. The concern for equity in health. *Journal of Epidemiology and Community Health,* 2002, 56:485–487.

115. *Road map for a health justice majority.* Oakland, CA, American Environics, 2006 (http://www.americanenvironics.com/PDF/Road_Map_for_Health_Justice_Majority_AE.pdf, accessed 1 July 2008).

116. Welzel I. A human development view on value change trends (1981–2006). *World Value Surveys,* 2007 (http://www.worldvaluessurvey.org/, accessed on 1 July 2008).

117. World values surveys database. Madrid, World Value Surveys, 2008 (http://www.worldvaluessurvey.com, accessed 2 July 2008).

118. *A global look at public perceptions of health problems, priorities and donors: the Kaiser/Pew global health survey.* Kaiser Family Foundation, December 2007 (http://www.kff.org/kaiserpolls/upload/7716.pdf , accessed 1 July 2008).

119. Blumenthal D, Hsiao W. Privatization and its discontents – the evolving Chinese health care system. *New England Journal of Medicine,* 2005, 353:1165–1170.

120. Lübker M. Globalization and perceptions of social inequality. *International Labour Review,* 2004, 143:191.

121. Taylor, B, Thomson, K. *Understanding change in social attitudes.* Aldershot, England, Dartmouth Publishing, 1996.

122. Gajdos T, Lhommeau B. L'attitude à l'égard des inegalités en France à la lumière du système de prélèvement socio-fiscal. Mai 1999 (http://thibault.gajdos.free.fr/pdf/cserc.pdf, accessed 2 July 2008).

123. Halman L et al. *Changing values and beliefs in 85 countries. Trends from the values surveys from 1981 to 2004.* Leiden and Boston, Brill, 2008 (European values studies 11; http://www.worldvaluessurvey.org/, accessed 2 July 2008).

124. De Maeseneer J et al. *Primary health care as a strategy for achieving equitable care: a literature review commissioned by the Health Systems Knowledge Network.* Geneva, World Health Organization, Commission on the Social Determinants of Health, 2007.

125. Burström K, Johannesson M, DIdericksen E. Increasing socio-economic inequalities in life expectancy and QALYs in Sweden 1980-1997. *Health Economics,* 2005, 14:831–850.

126. Marmot M. Achieving health equity: from root causes to fair outcomes. *Lancet,* 2007, 370:1153–1163.

127. *Health care: the stories we tell. Framing review.* Oakland CA, American Environics, 2006 (http.www.americanenvironics.com, accessed 2 July 2008).

128. Garland M, Oliver J. *Oregon health values survey 2004.* Tualatin, Oregon Health Decisions, 2004.

129. Mullan F, Frehywot S. Non-physician clinicians in 47 sub-Saharan African countries. *Lancet,* 2007, 370:2158–2163.

130. Koblinsky M et al. Going to scale with professional skilled care. *Lancet,* 2006, 368:1377–1386.

131. Lehmann U, Sanders D. *Community health workers: what do we know about them? The state of the evidence on programmes, activities, costs and impact on health outcomes of using community health workers.* Geneva, World Health Organization, Department of Human Resources for Health, Evidence and Information for Policy, 2007.

132. Dossyns P, Van Lerberghe W. The weakest link: competence and prestige as constraints to referral by isolated nurses in rural Niger. *Human Resources for Health,* 2004, 2:1–8.

133. Cheragi-Sohi S et al. What are the key attributes of primary care for patients? Building a conceptual map of patient preferences. *Health Expect,* 2006, 9:275–284.

134. Pongsupap Y, Van Lerberghe W. Choosing between public and private or between hospital and primary care? Responsiveness, patient-centredness and prescribing patterns in outpatient consultations in Bangkok. *Tropical Medicine & International Health,* 2006, 11:81–89.

135. Allen J et al. *The European definition of general practice/family practice.* Ljubljana, European Society of General Practice/Family Medicine, 2002 (http://www.globalfamilydoctor.com/publications/Euro_Def.pdf/, accessed 21 July 2008).

136. Gostin LO. Public health law in a new century. Part I: law as a tool to advance the community's health. *Journal of the American Medical Association,* 2000, 283:2837–2841.

137. Canadian Public Health Association and Welfare Canada and the World Health Organization. *Ottawa Charter for Health Promotion. First International Conference on Health Promotion, Ottawa, 17–21 November 1986.* Geneva, Department of Human Resources for Health, World Health Organization, 1986 (WHO/HPR/HEP/95.1; http://www.who.int/hpr/NPH/docs/ottawa_charter_hp.pdf, accessed 2 July 2008).

138. Kickbusch I. The contribution of the World Health Organization to a new public health and health promotion. *American Journal of Public Health,* 2003, 93:3.

139. Jaffré Y, Olivier de Sardan JP. *Une médecine inhospitalière.* Paris, APAD-Karthala (Hommes et sociétés), 2003.

140. Blank RH. *The price of life: the future of American health care.* New York, Colombia University Press, 1997.

141. Weissert C, Weissert W. *Governing health: the politics of health policy.* Baltimore MD, Johns Hopkins University Press, 2006.

142. Millenson ML. How the US news media made patient safety a priority. *BMJ,* 2002. 324:1044.

143. Davies H. Falling public trust in health services: Implications for accountability. *Journal of Health Services Research and Policy,* 1999, 4:193–194.

144. Gilson L. Trust and the development of health care as a social institution. *Social Science and Medicine,* 2003, 56:1453–1468.

145. Nutley S, Smith PC. League tables for performance improvement in health care. *Journal of Health Services & Research Policy,* 1998, 3:50–57.

146. Allsop J, Baggott R, Jones K. Health consumer groups and the national policy process. In: Henderson S, Petersen AR, eds. *Consuming health: the commodification of health care,* London, Routledge, 2002.

147. Rao H. Caveat emptor: the construction of non-profit consumer watchdog organizations. *American Journal of Sociology,* 1998, 103:912–961.

148. Larkin M. Public health watchdog embraces the web. *Lancet,* 2000, 356:1283–1283.

149. Lee K. Globalisation and the need for a strong public health response. *The European Journal of Public Health,* 1999 9:249–250.

150. McKee M, Figueras J. Setting priorities: can Britain learn from Sweden? *British Medical Journal,* 1996, 312:691–694.

151. Daniels N. Accountability for reasonableness. Establishing a fair process for priority setting is easier than agreeing on principles. *BMJ,* 2000, 321:1300–1301.

152. Martin D. Fairness, accountability for reasonableness, and the views of priority setting decision-makers. *Health Policy,* 2002, 61:279–290.

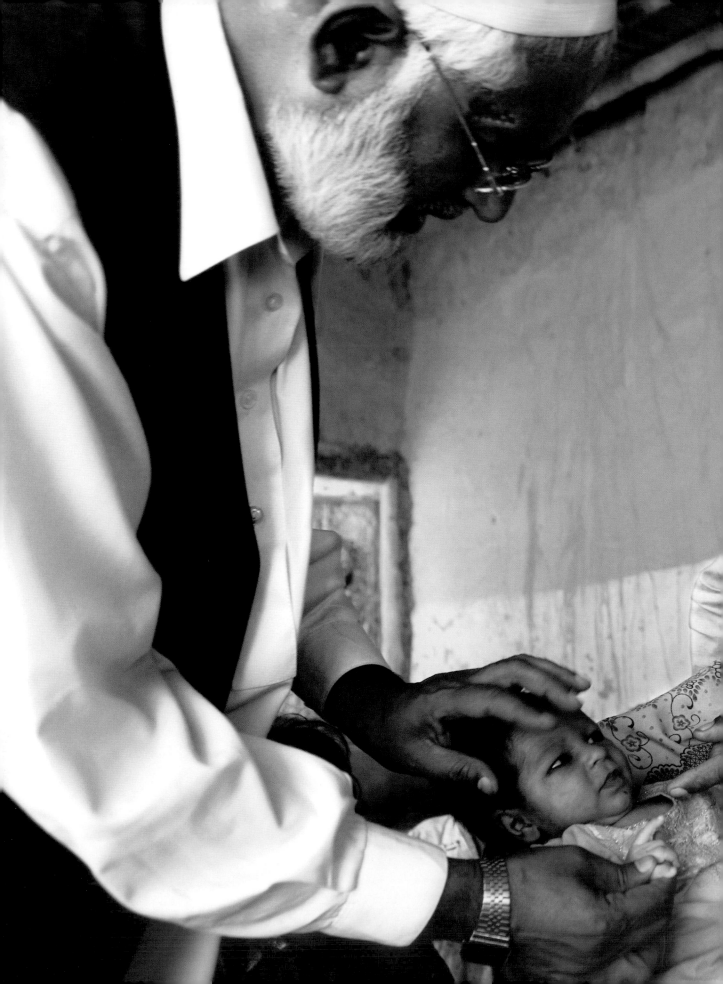

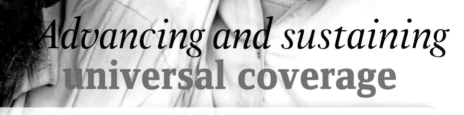

Advancing and sustaining universal coverage

People expect their health systems to be equitable. The roots of health inequities lie in social conditions outside the health system's direct control. These root causes have to be tackled through intersectoral and cross-government action. At the same time, the health sector can take significant actions to advance health equity internally. The basis for this is the set of reforms that aim at moving towards universal coverage, i.e. towards universal access to health services with social health protection.

The central place of health equity in PHC

"If you get sick, you have to choose: you either go without treatment or you lose the farm."[1] Nearly a century ago, the unforgiving reality of life in rural Canada prompted Matthew Anderson (1882–1974) to launch a tax-based health insurance scheme that eventually led to countrywide adoption of universal health care across Canada in 1965. Unfortunately, equally shocking lose-lose situations abound today across the world. More than 30 years after the clarion call of Alma-Ata for greater equity in health, most of the world's health-care systems continue to rely on the most inequitable method for financing health-care services: out-of-pocket payments by the sick or their families at the point of service. For 5.6 billion people in low- and middle-income countries, over half of all health-care expenditure is through out-of-pocket payments. This deprives many families of needed care because they cannot afford it. Also, more than 100 million people around the world are pushed into poverty each year because of catastrophic health-care expenditures[2]. There is a wealth of evidence demonstrating that financial protection is better, and catastrophic expenditure less frequent, in those countries in which there is more pre-payment for health care and less out-of-pocket payment. Conversely, catastrophic expenditure is more frequent when health care has to be paid for out-of-pocket at the point of service (Figure 2.1).

While equity marks one of PHC's boldest features, it is one of the areas where results have been most uneven and where the premium for more effective reforms is perhaps the greatest. Out-of-pocket payments for health care are but one of the sources of health inequity. Deeply unequal opportunities for health combined with endemic inequalities in health care provision lead to pervasive inequities in health outcomes[3]. Growing awareness of these regressive patterns is causing increasing intolerance of the whole spectrum of unnecessary, avoidable and unfair differences in health[4].

The extent of health inequities is documented in much more detail today. They stem from social stratification and political inequalities that lie outside the boundaries of the health system. Income and social status matter, as do the neighbourhoods where people live, their employment conditions and factors, such as personal behaviour, race and stress[5]. Health inequities also find their roots in the way health systems exclude people, such as inequities in availability, access, quality and burden of payment, and even in the way clinical practice is conducted[6]. Left to their own devices, health systems do not move towards greater equity. Most health services – hospitals in particular, but also first-level care – are consistently inequitable providing more and higher quality services to the well-off than to the poor, who are in greater need[7,8,9,10]. Differences in vulnerability and exposure combine with inequalities in health care to lead to unequal health outcomes; the latter further contribute to the social stratification that led to the inequalities in the first place. People are rarely indifferent to this cycle of inequalities, making their concerns as relevant to politicians as they are to health-system managers.

It takes a wide range of interventions to tackle the social determinants of health and make health systems contribute to more health equity[11]. These interventions reach well beyond the traditional realm of health-service policies, relying on the mobilization of stakeholders and constituencies outside the health sector[12]. They include[13]:

■ reduction of social stratification, e.g. by reducing income inequality through taxes and subsidized public services, providing jobs with

Figure 2.1 Catastrophic expenditure related to out-of-pocket payment at the point of service[1]

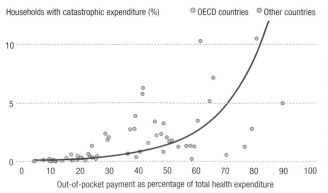

adequate pay, using labour intensive growth strategies, promoting equal opportunities for women and making free education available, etc.;

- reduction of vulnerabilities, e.g. by providing social security for the unemployed or disabled, developing social networks at community level, introducing social inclusion policies and policies that protect mothers while working or studying, offering cash benefits or transfers, providing free healthy lunches at school, etc.;
- protection, particularly of the disadvantaged, against exposure to health hazards, e.g. by introducing safety regulations for the physical and social environment, providing safe water and sanitation, promoting healthy lifestyles, establishing healthy housing policies, etc.);
- mitigation of the consequences of unequal health outcomes that contribute to further social stratification, e.g. by protecting the sick from unfair dismissal from their jobs.

The need for such multiple strategies could discourage some health leaders who might feel that health inequality is a societal problem over which they have little influence. Yet, they do have a responsibility to address health inequality. The policy choices they make for the health sector define the extent to which health systems exacerbate or mitigate health inequalities and their capacity to mobilize around the equity agenda within government and civil society. These choices also play a key part in society's response to citizens' aspirations for more equity and solidarity. The question, therefore, is not if, but how health leaders can more effectively pursue strategies that will build greater equity in the provision of health services.

Moving towards universal coverage

The fundamental step a country can take to promote health equity is to move towards universal coverage: universal access to the full range of personal and non-personal health services they need, with social health protection. Whether the arrangements for universal coverage are tax-based or are organized through social health insurance, or a mix of both, the principles are the same: pooling pre-paid contributions collected on the basis of ability to pay, and using these funds to ensure that services are available, accessible and produce quality care for those who need them, without exposing them to the risk of catastrophic expenditures[14,15,16]. Universal coverage is not, by itself, sufficient to ensure health for all and health equity – inequalities persist in countries with universal or near-universal coverage – but it provides the necessary foundation[9].

While universal coverage is fundamental to building health equity, it has rarely been the object of an easy social consensus. Indeed, in countries where universal coverage has been achieved or embraced as a political goal, the idea has often met with strong initial resistance, for example, from associations of medical professionals concerned about the impact of government-managed health insurance schemes on their incomes and working conditions, or from financial experts determined to rein in public spending. As with other entitlements that are now taken for granted in almost all high-income countries, universal health coverage has generally been struggled for and won by social movements, not spontaneously bestowed by political leaders. There is now widespread consensus that providing such coverage is simply part of the package of core obligations that any legitimate government must fulfil vis-à-vis its citizens. In itself, this is a political achievement that shapes the modernization of society.

Industrialized countries, particularly in Europe, began to put social health protection schemes in place in the late 19th century, moving towards universalism in the second half of the 20th century. The opportunity now exists for low- and middle-income countries to implement comparable approaches. Costa Rica, Mexico, the Rebublic of Korea, Thailand and Turkey are among the countries that have already introduced ambitious universal coverage schemes, moving significantly faster than industrialized countries did in the past. Other countries are weighing similar options[14]. The technical challenge of moving towards universal coverage is to expand coverage in three ways (Figure 2.2).

The breadth of coverage – the proportion of the population that enjoys social health protection – must expand progressively to encompass

Figure 2.2 Three ways of moving towards universal coverage[17]

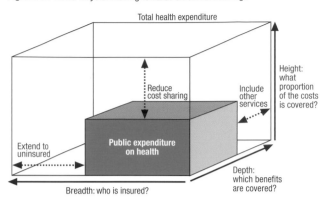

Meanwhile, the *depth of coverage* must also grow, expanding the range of essential services that are necessary to address people's health needs effectively, taking into account demand and expectations, and the resources society is willing and able to allocate to health. The determination of the corresponding "essential package" of benefits can play a key role here, provided the process is conducted appropriately (Box 2.2).

The third dimension, *the height of coverage*, i.e. the portion of health-care costs covered through pooling and pre-payment mechanisms must also rise, diminishing reliance on out-of-pocket co-payments at the point of service delivery. In the 1980s and 1990s, many countries introduced user fees in an effort to infuse new resources into struggling services, often in a context of disengagement of the state and dwindling public resources for health. Most undertook these measures without anticipating the extent of the damage they would do. In many settings, dramatic declines in service use ensued, particularly among vulnerable groups[20], while the frequency of catastrophic expenditure increased. Some countries have since reconsidered their position and have started phasing out user fees and replacing the lost income from pooled funds (government subsidies or contracts, insurance

the uninsured, i.e. the population groups that lack access to services and/or social protection against the financial consequences of taking up health care. Expanding the breadth of coverage is a complex process of progressive expansion and merging of coverage models (Box 2.1). During this process, care must be taken to ensure safety nets for the poorest and most vulnerable until they also are covered. It may take years to cover the entire population but, as recent experience from a number of middle-income countries shows, it is possible to move much faster than was the case for industrialized countries during the 20th century.

Box 2.1 Best practices in moving towards universal coverage

Emphasize pre-payment from the start. It may take many years before access to health services and financial protection against the costs involved in their use are available for all: it took Japan and the United Kingdom 36 years[14]. The road may seem discouragingly long, particularly for the poorest countries, where health-care networks are sparsely developed, financial protection schemes embryonic and the health sector highly dependent on external funds. Particularly in these countries, however, it is crucial to move towards pre-payment systems from a very early stage and to resist the temptation to rely on user fees. Setting up and maintaining appropriate mechanisms for pre-payment builds the institutional capacity to manage the financing of the system along with the extension of service supply that is usually lacking in such contexts.

Coordinate funding sources. In order to organize universal coverage, it is necessary to consider all sources of funding in a country: public, private, external and domestic. In low-income countries, it is particularly important that international funding be channelled through nascent pre-payment and pooling schemes and institutions rather than through project or programme funding. Routing funds in this way has two purposes. It makes external funding more stable and predictable and helps build the institutional capacity to develop and extend supply, access and financial protection in a balanced way.

Combine schemes to build towards full coverage. Many countries with limited resources and administrative capacity have experimented with a multitude of voluntary insurance schemes: community, cooperative, employer-based and other private schemes, as a way to foster pre-payment and pooling in preparation for the move towards more comprehensive national systems[18]. Such schemes are no substitute for universal coverage although they can become building blocks of the universal system[18]. Realizing universal coverage means coordinating or combining these schemes progressively into a coherent whole that ensures coverage to all population groups[15] and builds bridges with broader social protection programmes[19].

Box 2.2 Defining "essential packages": what needs to be done to go beyond a paper exercise?

In recent years, many low- and midde-income countries (55 out of a sample of 69 reviewed in 2007) have gone through exercises to define the package of benefits they feel should be available to all their citizens. This has been one of the key strategies in improving the effectiveness of health systems and the equitable distribution of resources. It is supposed to make priority setting, rationing of care, and trade-offs between breadth and depth of coverage explicit.

On the whole, attempts to rationalize service delivery by defining packages have not been particularly successful[24]. In most cases, their scope has been limited to maternal and child health care, and to health problems considered as global health priorities. The lack of attention, for example, to chronic and noncommunicable diseases confirms the under-valuation of the demographic and epidemiological transitions and the lack of consideration for perceived needs and demand. The packages rarely give guidance on the division of tasks and responsibilities, or on the defining features of primary care, such as comprehensiveness, continuity or person-centredness.

A more sophisticated approach is required to make the definition of benefit packages more relevant. The way Chile has provided a detailed specification of the health rights of its citizens[25] suggests a number of principles of good practice.

- The exercise should not be limited to a set of predefined priorities: it should look at demand as well as at the full range of health needs.
- It should specify what should be provided at primary and secondary levels.
- The implementation of the package should be costed so that political decision-makers are aware of what will *not* be included if health care remains under-funded.
- There have to be institutionalized mechanisms for evidence-based review of the package of benefits.
- People need to be informed about the benefits they can claim, with mechanisms of mediation when claims are being denied. Chile went to great lengths to ensure that the package of benefits corresponds to people's expectations, with studies, surveys and systems to capture the complaints and misgivings of users[26].

or pre-payment schemes)[21]. This has resulted in substantial increases in the use of services, especially by the poor[20]. In Uganda, for example, service use increased suddenly and dramatically and the increase was sustained after the elimination of user fees (Figure 2.3)[22,23].

Pre-payment and pooling institutionalizes solidarity between the rich and the less well-off, and between the healthy and the sick. It lifts barriers to the uptake of services and reduces the risk that people will incur catastrophic expenses when they are sick. Finally, it provides the means to re-invest in the availability, range and quality of services.

Challenges in moving towards universal coverage

All universal coverage reforms have to find compromises between the speed with which they increase coverage and the breadth, depth and height of coverage. However, the way countries devise their strategies and focus their reforms very much depends on their specific national contexts.

In some countries, a very large part of the population lives in extremely deprived areas, with an absent or dysfunctional health-care infrastructure. These are countries of mass exclusion typically brought to mind when one talks about "scaling up": the poor and remote rural areas where health-care networks have not been deployed yet or where, after years of neglect, the health infrastructure continues to exist in name only. Such patterns occur in low-income countries

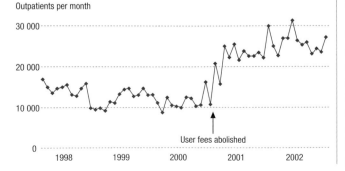

Figure 2.3 Impact of abolishing user fees on outpatient attendance in Kisoro district, Uganda: outpatient attendance 1998–2002[23]

Outpatients per month

User fees abolished

such as Bangladesh, Chad and Niger (Figure 2.4), and are common in conflict and post-conflict areas where health workers have departed and the health infrastructure has been destroyed and needs to be rebuilt from scratch.

In other parts of the world, the challenge is in providing health support to widely dispersed populations, for example, in small island states, remote desert or mountainous regions, and among nomadic and some indigenous populations. Ensuring access to quality care in these settings entails grappling with the diseconomies of scale connected with small, scattered populations; logistical constraints on referral; difficulties linked to limited infrastructure and communications capacities; and, in some cases, more specific technical complications, such as maintaining patient records for nomadic groups.

A different challenge is extending coverage in settings where inequalities do not result from the lack of available health infrastructure, but from the way health care is organized, regulated and, above all, paid for by official or under-the-counter user charges. These are situations where under-utilization of available services is concentrated among the poor, whereas users are exposed to the risks of catastrophic expenditure. Such patterns of exclusion occur in countries such as Colombia, Nicaragua and Turkey (Figure 2.4). It is particularly striking in the many urban areas of low- and middle-income countries where a plethora of assorted, unregulated, commercial health-care providers charge users prohibitive fees while providing inadequate services.

Ways of tackling the situations described in this section are elaborated below.

Rolling out primary-care networks to fill the availability gap

In areas where no health services are available for large population groups, or where such services are grossly inadequate or fragmented, the basic health-care infrastructure needs to be built or rebuilt, often from the ground up. These areas are always severely resource-constrained and frequently affected by conflicts or complex emergencies, while the scale of under-servicing, also in other sectors, engenders logistical difficulties and problems in deploying health professionals. Health planners in these settings face a fundamental strategic dilemma: whether to prioritize a massive scale-up of a limited set of interventions to the entire population or a progressive roll-out of more comprehensive primary-care systems on a district-by-district basis.

Some would advocate, in the name of speed and equity, an approach in which a restricted number of priority programmes is rolled out simultaneously to all the inhabitants in the deprived areas. This allows for task shifting to low-skilled personnel, lay workers and volunteers and, consequently, rapid extension of coverage. It is still central to what the global community often prescribes for the rural areas of the poorest countries[28], and quite a number of countries have chosen this option over the last 30 years. Ethiopia, for example, is currently deploying 30 000 health extension workers to provide massive numbers of people with a limited package of priority preventive interventions. The poor skills base is often well recognized as a limiting factor[29], but Ethiopia's extension workers are no longer as low skilled as they once were, and currently benefit from a year of post-Grade 10 training. Nevertheless, skill limitations reinforce the focus on a limited number of effective but simple interventions.

Scaling up a limited number of interventions has the advantage of rapidly covering the entire population and focusing resources on what is known to be cost effective. The downside is that

Figure 2.4 Different patterns of exclusion: massive deprivation in some countries, marginalization of the poor in others. Births attended by medically trained personnel (percentage), by income group[27]

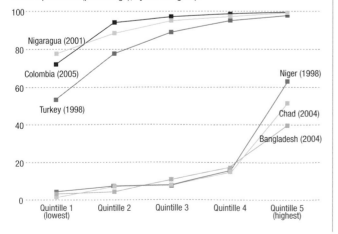

when people experience health problems, they want them to be dealt with, whether or not they fit nicely within the programmatic priorities that are being proposed. Ignoring this dimension of demand too much opens the door to "drug peddlers", "injectors" and other types of providers, who can capitalize on commercial opportunities arising from unmet health needs. They offer patients an appealing alternative, but one that is often exploitative and harmful. Compared with a situation of utter lack of health action, there is an indisputable benefit in scaling up even a very limited package of interventions and the possibility of relying on low-skilled staff makes it an attractive option. However, upgrading often proves more difficult than initially envisaged[30] and, in the meantime, valuable time, resources and credibility are lost which might have allowed for investment in a more ambitious, but also more sustainable and effective primary-care infrastructure.

The alternative is a progressive roll-out of primary care, district-by-district, of a network of health centres with the necessary hospital support. Such a response obviously includes the priority interventions, but integrated in a comprehensive primary-care package. The extension platform is the primary-care centre: a professionalized infrastructure where the interface with the community is organized, with a problem solving capacity and modular expansion of the range of activities. The Islamic Republic of Iran's progressive roll-out of rural coverage is an impressive example of this model. As one of the fathers of the country's PHC strategy put it: "Since it was impossible to launch the project in all provinces at the same time, we decided to focus on a single province each year" (Box 2.3).

The limiting factors for a progressive roll-out of primary-care networks are the lack of a stable cadre of mid-level staff with the leadership qualities to organize health districts and with the ability to maintain, over the years, the constant effort required to build sustainable results for the entire population. Where the roll-out has been conducted as an administrative exercise, it has led to disappointment: many health districts exist in name only. But where impatience and pressure for short-term visibility has been managed

---

Box 2.3 Closing the urban-rural gap through progressive expansion of PHC coverage in rural areas in the Islamic Republic of Iran[31]

In the 1970s, the Iranian Government's policies emphasized prevention as a long-term investment, allocation of resources to rural and under-privileged areas, and prioritizing ambulatory care over hospitalization. A network of district teams to manage and oversee almost 2500 village-based rural health centres was established. These centres are staffed by a team that includes a general practitioner, midwife, nurse and several health technicians. Each of the rural health centres oversees 1–5 smaller points of care known as "health houses". With 17 000 of these health houses, over 90% of the rural population has access to health care. In remote rural areas, these health houses are staffed by *Behvarz* (multi-purpose health workers) who are selected by the community, receive between 12 and 18 months training and are then recruited by the Government. The district teams provide training based on problem-solving, as well as ongoing supervision and support.

The Government deployed this strategy progressively, extending coverage to one province at a time. Over the years, the PHC network has grown and is now able to provide services to over 24 million people in rural villages and small cities by bringing the points of care closer to where people live and work, as well as by training the necessary auxiliary health staff to provide family planning, preventive care services, and essential curative care for the majority of health problems. Rural health service utilization rates are now the same as in urban areas. The progressive roll-out of this system has helped to reduce the urban-rural gap in child mortality (Figure 2.5).

Figure 2.5 Under-five mortality in rural and urban areas, the Islamic Republic of Iran, 1980–2000[32]

Mortality per 1000 children under five

adequately, a blend of response to need and demand, and participation of the population and key actors has made it possible to build robust primary-care networks, even in very difficult and resource-constrained settings of conflict, and post-conflict environments (Box 2.4).

The distinction between rapid deployment of priority interventions and progressive roll-out of primary-care networks is, in practice, often not as straightforward as described above. However, for all the convergence, trying to balance speed and sustainability is a real political dilemma[30]. Mali, among others, has shown that, given the choice, people willingly opt for progressive roll-out, making community health centres – whose infrastructure is owned and personnel employed by the local community – the basis of functional health districts.

Crucially, concern for equity should not be translated into a "lowest common denominator" approach: equal access for all to a set of largely unsatisfactory services. Quality and sustainability are important, particularly since nowadays the multitude of varied and dynamic governmental, not-for-profit and for-profit private providers of various kinds are in dire need of alignment. Progressive roll-out of health services provides the opportunity to establish welcome leadership coherence in health-care provision at district level. Typical large-scale examples of this approach in developing countries are the contracting out of district health services in Cambodia, or the incorporation of missionary "designated district hospitals" in East Africa. Nevertheless, there is no getting away from the need for massive and sustained investment to expand and maintain health districts in the long term and from the fact that this represents a considerable challenge in a context of sluggish economic growth and stagnating health expenditure.

Extending health-care networks to underserved areas depends on public initiative and incentives. One way to accelerate the extension of coverage is to adjust budget allocation formulae (or contract specifications) to reflect the extra efforts required to contact hard-to-reach populations. Several countries have taken steps in this direction. In January 2004, for example, the United Republic of Tanzania adopted a revised formula for the allocation of basket funds to districts that includes population size and under-five mortality as a proxy for disease burden and poverty level, while adjusting for the differential costs of providing health services in rural and low-density areas. Similarly, allocations to districts under Uganda's PHC budget factor in the districts' Human Development Index and levels of external health funding, in addition to population size. Supplements are paid to districts with difficult security situations or lacking a district hospital[20]. In Chile, budgets are allocated on a capitation basis but, as part of the PHC reforms, these were adjusted using municipal human development indices and a factor to reflect the isolation of underserved areas.

Overcoming the isolation of dispersed populations

Although providing access to services for dispersed populations is often a daunting logistical challenge, some countries have dealt with it by developing creative approaches. Devising mechanisms to share innovative experiences and results has clearly been a key step, for example, through the "Healthy Islands" initiative, launched at the meeting of Ministers and Heads of Health in Yanuca, Fiji, in 1995[34]. The initiative brings together health policy-makers and practitioners to address challenges to islanders' health and well-being from an explicitly multi-sectoral perspective, with a focus on expanding coverage of curative health-care services, but also reinforcing promotive strategies and cross-sectoral action on the determinants of health and health equity.

Through the Healthy Islands initiative and related experiences, a number of principles have emerged as crucial to the advancement of universal coverage in these settings. The first concerns collaboration in organizing infrastructure that maximizes scales of efficiency. An isolated community may be unable to afford key inputs to expand coverage, which includes infrastructure, technologies and human resources (particularly the training of personnel). However, when communities join forces, they can secure such inputs at manageable costs[35]. A second strategic focus is on "mobile resources" or those that can overcome distance and geographical obstacles efficiently and affordably. Depending on the setting, this strategic focus may include transportation, radio communications, and other information and communications technologies. Telecommunications

---

Box 2.4 The robustness of PHC-led health systems: 20 years of expanding performance in Rutshuru, the Democratic Republic of the Congo

Rutshuru is a health district in the east of the country. It has a network of health centres, a referral hospital and a district management team where community participation has been fostered for years through local committees. Rutshuru has experienced severe stress over the years, testing the robustness of the district health system.

Over the last 30 years, the economy of the country has gone into a sharp decline. GDP dropped from US$ 300 per capita in the 1980s to below US$ 100 at the end of the 1990s. Massive impoverishment was made worse as the State retreated from the health sector. This was compounded by an interruption of overseas development aid in the early 1990s. In that context, Rutshuru suffered inter-ethnic strife, a massive influx of refugees and two successive wars. This complex of disasters severely affected the working conditions of health professionals and access to health services for the 200 000 people living in the district.

Nevertheless, instead of collapsing, PHC services continued their expansion over the years. The number of health centres and their output increased (Figure 2.6), and quality of care improved for acute cases (case-fatality rate after caesarean section dropped from 7% to less than 3%) as well as for chronic patients (at least 60% of tuberculosis patients were treated successfully). With no more than 70 nurses and three medical doctors at a time, and in the midst of war and havoc, the health centres and the district hospital took care of more than 1 500 000 disease episodes in 20 years, immunized more than 100 000 infants, provided midwifery care to 70 000 women and carried out 8 000 surgical procedures. This shows that, even in disastrous circumstances, a robust district health system can improve health-care outputs.

These results were achieved with modest means. Out-of-pocket payments amounted to US$ 0.5 per capita per year. Nongovernmental organizations subsidized the district with an average of US$ 1.5 per capita per year. The Government's contribution was virtually nil during most of these 20 years. The continuity of the work under extremely difficult circumstances can be explained by team work and collegial decision-making, unrelenting efforts to build up and maintain a critical mass of dedicated human resources, and limited but constant nongovernmental support, which provided a minimum of resources for health facilities and gave the district management team the opportunity to maintain contact with the outside world.

Three lessons can be learnt from this experience. In the long run, PHC-led health districts are an organizational model that has the robustness to resist extremely adverse conditions. Maintaining minimal financial support and supervision to such districts can yield very significant results, while empowering and retaining national health professionals. Local health services have a considerable potential for coping with crises[33].

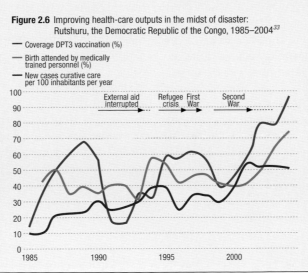

Figure 2.6 Improving health-care outputs in the midst of disaster: Rutshuru, the Democratic Republic of the Congo, 1985–2004[33]

— Coverage DPT3 vaccination (%)
— Birth attended by medically trained personnel (%)
— New cases curative care per 100 inhabitants per year

---

can enable less skilled frontline health-centre staff to be advised and guided by experts at a distance in real time[36]. Finally, the financing of health care for dispersed populations poses specific challenges, which often require larger per capita expenditure compared to more clustered populations. In countries whose territories include both high-density and low-density populations, it is expected that dispersed populations will receive some subsidy of care. After all, equity does not come without solidarity.

Providing alternatives to unregulated commercial services

In urban and periurban contexts, health services are physically within reach of the poor and other vulnerable populations. The presence of multiple health-care providers does not mean, however, that these groups are protected from diseases, nor that they can get quality care when they need it: the more privileged tend to get better access to the best services, public and private, easily coming out on top in a *de facto* competition for scarce resources. In the urban and increasingly in the rural areas of many low- and middle-income countries – from India and Viet Nam to sub-Saharan Africa – much health care for the poor is provided by small-scale, largely unregulated and often unlicenced providers, both commercial and not-for-profit. Often, they work alongside dysfunctional public services and capture an overwhelmingly large part of the health-care market, while the health promotion and prevention agenda is totally ignored. Vested interests make the promotion of universal coverage paradoxically more difficult in these circumstances than in areas where the challenge is to build health-care delivery networks from scratch.

These contexts often combine problems of financial exploitation, bad quality and unsafe care, and exclusion from needed services[37,38,39,40,41,42,43,44,45,46]. The Pan American Health Organization (PAHO) has estimated that 47% of Latin America's population is excluded from needed services[47]. This may be for broader reasons of poverty, ethnicity or gender, or because the resources of the health system are not correctly targeted. It may be because there are no adequate systems to protect people against catastrophic expenditure or from financial exploitation by unscrupulous or insensitive providers. It may have to do with the way people, rightly or wrongly, perceive health services: lack of trust, the expectation of ill-treatment or discrimination, uncertainty about the cost-of-care, or the anticipation that the cost will be unaffordable or catastrophic. Services may also be untimely, ineffective, unresponsive or plain discriminatory, providing poorer patients with inferior treatment[48,49,21]. As a result, health outcomes vary considerably by social class, even in well-regulated and well-funded health-care systems.

In addressing these patterns of exclusion within the health-care sector, the starting point is to create or strengthen networks of accessible quality primary-care services that rely on pooled pre-payment or public resources for their funding. Whether these networks are expanded by contracting commercial or not-for-profit providers, or by revitalizing dysfunctional public facilities is not the critical issue. The point is to ensure that they offer care of an acceptable standard. A critical mass of primary-care centres that provide an essential package of quality services free-of-charge, provides an important alternative to sub-standard, exploitative commercial care. Furthermore, peer pressure and consumer demand can help to create an environment in which regulation of the commercial sector becomes possible. More active involvement of municipal authorities in pre-payment and pooling schemes to improve the supply of quality care is probably one of the avenues to follow, particularly where ministries of health with budgetary constraints also have to extend services to underserved rural areas.

Targeted interventions to complement universal coverage mechanisms

Rising average national income, a growing supply of health-care providers and accelerated progress towards universal coverage are, unfortunately, not sufficient to eliminate health inequities. Socially determined health differences among population groups persist in high-income countries with robust, universal health-care and social-service systems, such as Finland and France[11,50]. Health inequalities do not just exist between the poor and the non-poor, but across the entire socioeconomic gradient. There are circumstances where other forms of exclusion are of prime concern, including the exclusion of adolescents, ethnic groups, drug users and those affected by stigmatizing diseases[51]. In Australia, Canada and New Zealand, among others, health equity gaps between Aboriginal and non-Aboriginal populations have emerged as national political issues[52,53,54]. In other settings, inequalities in women's access to health care merit attention[55]. In the United States, for example, declines in female life expectancy of up to five years in over 1000 counties point to differential exposure and clustering of risks to health even as the country's economy and health sector continues to grow[56]. For a variety of reasons, some groups within these societies are either not reached or insufficiently reached by opportunities for health or services and continue to experience health outcomes systematically inferior to those of more advantaged groups.

Thus, it is necessary to embed universal coverage in wider social protection schemes and to complement it with specially designed, targeted forms of outreach to vulnerable and excluded groups[57]. Established health-care networks often do not make all possible efforts to ensure that everyone in their target population has access to the full range of health benefits they need, as this requires extra efforts, such as home visits, outreach services, specialized language and cultural facilitation, evening consultations, etc. These may, however, mitigate the effect of social stratification and inequalities in the uptake of services[58]. They may also offer the opportunity to construct comprehensive support packages to foster social inclusion of historically marginalized populations, in collaboration with other government sectors and with affected communities. Chile's *Chile Solidario* (Chilean Solidarity) model of outreach to families in long-term poverty is one example (Box 2.5)[59]. Such targeted measures may include subsidizing people – not services – to take up specific health services, for example, through vouchers[60,61] for maternal care as in India and Yemen, for bednets as in the United Republic of Tanzania[62,63], for contraceptive uptake by adolescents[64] or care for the elderly uninsured as in the United States[65]. Conditional cash transfers, where the beneficiary is not only enabled, but compelled to take up services is another model, which has been introduced in several countries in

Latin America. A recent systematic review of six such programmes suggests that conditional cash transfers can be effective in increasing the use of preventive services and improving nutritional and anthropometric outcomes, sometimes improving health status[66]. However, their overall effect on health status remains less clear and so does their comparative advantage over traditional, unconditional, income maintenance, through universal entitlements, social insurance or – less-effective – means-tested social assistance.

Targeted measures are not substitutes for the long-term drive towards universal coverage. They can be useful and necessary complements, but without simultaneous institutionalization of the financing models and system structures that support universal coverage, targeted approaches are unlikely to overcome the inequalities generated by socioeconomic stratification and exclusion. This is all the more important since systematic evaluation of methods to target the excluded is scarce and marred by the limited number of documented experiences and a bias towards reporting preferentially on successful pilots[67]. If anything definite can be said today, it is that the strategies for reaching the unreached will have to be multiple and contextualized, and that no single targeting measure will suffice to correct health inequalities effectively, certainly not in the absence of a universal coverage policy.

Box 2.5 Targeting social protection in Chile[59]

Established by law, the Chilean social protection programme (*Chile Solidario*) involves three main components to improve conditions for people living in extreme poverty: direct psycho-social support, financial support and priority access to social programmes. The direct psycho-social support component involves families in extreme poverty being identified according to pre-defined criteria and invited to enter into an agreement with a designated social worker. The social worker assists them to build individual and family capacities that help them to strengthen their links with social networks and to gain access to the social benefits to which they are entitled. In addition to psycho-social support, there is also financial support in terms of cash transfers and pensions, as well as subsidies for raising families or covering water and sanitation costs. Finally, the social protection programme also provides preferential access to pre-school programmes, adult literacy courses, employment programmes and preventive health visits for women and children.

This social protection programme complements a multisectoral effort targeting all children aged 0–18 years (*Chile Crece Contigo* – Chile Grows with You). The aim is to promote early childhood development through pre-school education programmes, preventive health checks, improved parental leave and increased child benefits. Better access to child-care services is also included as is enforcing the right of working mothers to nurse their babies, which is designed to stimulate women's insertion into the employment market.

Mobilizing for health equity

Health systems are invariably inequitable. More and higher quality services gravitate to the well-off who need them less than the poor and marginalized[8]. The universal coverage reforms required to move towards greater equity demand the enduring commitment of the highest political levels of society. Two levers may be especially important in accelerating action on health equity and maintaining momentum over time. The first is raising the visibility of health inequities in public awareness and policy debates: the history of progress in the health of populations is intimately linked to the measurement of health inequalities. It was the observation of excess mortality among the working class that informed the "Great Sanitary Awakening" reforms of the Poor Laws Commission in the United Kingdom in the 1830s[68]. The second is the creation of space for civil society participation in shaping the PHC reforms that are to advance health equity: the history of progress in universal coverage is intimately linked to that of social movements.

Increasing the visibility of health inequities

With the economic optimism of the 1960s and 1970s (and the expansion of social insurance in industrialized countries), poverty ceased being a priority issue for many policy-makers. It took Alma-Ata to put equity back on the political agenda. The lack of systematic measurement and monitoring to translate this agenda into concrete challenges has long been a major constraint in advancing the PHC agenda. In recent years, income-related and other health inequalities have been studied in greater depth. The introduction of composite asset indices has made it possible to re-analyze demographic and health surveys from an equity viewpoint[69]. This has generated a wealth of documentary evidence on socioeconomic differentials in health outcomes and access to care. It took this acceleration of the measurement of poverty and inequalities, particularly since the mid-1990s, to bring first poverty and then, more generally, the challenge of persisting inequalities to the centre of the health policy debate.

Measurement of health inequities is paramount when confronting the common misperceptions that strongly influence health policy debates[70,71].

- Simple population averages are sufficient to assess progress – they are not.
- Health systems designed for universal access are equitable – they are a necessary, but not a sufficient condition.
- In poor countries, everybody is equally poor and equally unhealthy – all societies are stratified.
- The main concern is between countries' differences – inequalities within countries matter most to people.
- Well-intended reforms to improve efficiency will ultimately benefit everybody – they often have unintended inequitable consequences. Measurement matters for a variety of reasons[2].
- It is important to know the extent and understand the nature of health inequalities and exclusion in a given society, so as to be able to share that information and translate it into objectives for change.
- It is equally important, for the same reasons, to identify and understand the determinants of health inequality not only in general terms, but also within each specific national context. Health authorities must be informed of the extent to which current or planned health policies contribute to inequalities, so as to be able to correct them.
- Progress with reforms designed to reduce health inequalities, i.e. progress in moving towards universal coverage, needs to be monitored, so as to steer and correct these reforms as they unfold.

Despite policy-makers' long-held commitment to the value of equity in health, its definition and measurement represent a more recent public health science. Unless health information systems collect data using standardized social stratifiers, such as socioeconomic status, gender, ethnicity and geographical area, it is difficult to identify and locate inequalities and, unless their magnitude and nature are uncovered, it is unlikely that they will be adequately addressed[72]. The now widely available analyses of Demographic and Health Survey (DHS) data by asset quintiles have made a major difference in the awareness of policy-makers about health equity problems in their countries. There are also examples of how domestic capacities and capabilities can be strengthened to better understand and manage equity problems. For example, Chile has recently embarked on integrating health sector information systems in order to have more comprehensive information on determinants and to improve the ability to disaggregate information according to socioeconomic groups. Indonesia has added health modules to household expenditure and demographic surveys. Building in capabilities, across administrative database systems, to link health and socioeconomic data through unique identifiers (national insurance numbers or census geo-codes) is key to socioeconomic stratification and provides information that is usually inaccessible. However, this is more than a technical challenge. Measuring health systems' progress towards equity requires an explicit deliberative process to identify what constitutes a fair distribution of health against shortfalls and gaps that can be measured[73]. It relies on the development of institutional collaboration between multiple stakeholders to ensure that measurement and monitoring translates into concrete political proposals for better equity and solidarity.

Creating space for civil society participation and empowerment

Knowledge about health inequalities can only be translated into political proposals if there is organized social demand. Demand from the communities that bear the burden of existing inequities and other concerned groups in civil society are among the most powerful motors driving universal coverage reforms and efforts to reach the unreached and the excluded.

The amount of grassroots advocacy to improve the health and welfare of populations in need has grown enormously in the last 30 years, mostly within countries, but also globally. There are now thousands of groups around the world, large and small, local and global, calling for action to improve the health of particularly deprived social groups or those suffering from specific health conditions. These groups, which were virtually non-existent in the days of the Alma-Ata, constitute a powerful voice of collective action.

Box 2.6 Social policy in the city of Ghent, Belgium: how local authorities can support intersectoral collaboration between health and welfare organizations[76]

In 2004, a regional government decree in Flanders, Belgium, institutionalized the direct participation of local stakeholders and citizens in intersectoral collaboration on social rights. This now applies at the level of cities and villages in the region. In one of these cities, Ghent, some 450 local actors of the health and welfare sector have been clustered in 11 thematic forums: legal help; support and security of minors; services for young people and adolescents; child care; ethnic cultural minorities; people with a handicap; the elderly; housing; work and employment; people living on a "critical income"; and health.

The local authorities facilitate and support the collaboration of the various organizations and sectors, for example, through the collection and monitoring of data, information and communication, access to services, and efforts to make services more pro-active. They are also responsible for networking between all the sectors with a view to improving coordination. They pick up the signals, bottlenecks, proposals and plans, and are responsible for channelling them, if appropriate, to the province, region, federal state or the European Union for translation into relevant political decisions and legislation.

A steering committee reports directly to the city council and integrates the work of the 11 forums. The support of the administration and a permanent working party is critical for the sustainability and quality of the work in the different groups. Participation of all stakeholders is particularly prominent in the health forum: it includes local hospitals, family physicians, primary-care services, pharmacists, mental health facilities, self-help groups, home care, health promotion agencies, academia sector, psychiatric home care, and community health centres.

This complex web of collaboration is showing results. Intersectoral coordination contributes to a more efficient local social policy. For the period 2008–2013, four priority themes have been identified in a bottom-up process: sustainable housing, access to health care, reduced thresholds to social rights, and optimization of growth and development. The yearly action plan operationalizes the policy through improvement projects in areas that include financial access to health care, educational support, care for the homeless, and affordable and flexible child care. Among the concrete realizations is the creation of Ghent's "social house", a network of service entry points situated in the different neighbourhoods of the city, where delivery of primary care is organized with special attention to the most vulnerable groups of people. The participating organizations report that the creation of the sectoral forums, in conjunction with the organization of intersectoral cooperation, has significantly improved the way social determinants of health are tackled in the city.

The mobilization of groups and communities to address what they consider to be their most important health problems and health-related inequalities is a necessary complement to the more technocratic and top-down approach to assessing social inequalities and determining priorities for action.

Many of these groups have become capable lobbyists, for example, by gaining access to HIV/AIDS treatment, abolishing user fees and promoting universal coverage. However, these achievements should not mask the contributions that the direct engagement of affected communities and civil society organizations can have in eliminating sources of exclusion within local health services. Costa Rica's "bias-free framework" is one example among many. It has been used successfully to foster dialogue with and among members of vulnerable communities by uncovering local practices of exclusion and barriers to access not readily perceived by providers and by spurring action to address the underlying causes of ill-health. Concrete results, such as the reorganization of a maternity hospital around the people's needs and expectations can transcend the local dimension, as was the case in Costa Rica when local reorganization was used as a template for a national effort[74].

However, there is much the health system itself can do to mitigate the effects of social inequities and promote fairer access to health services at local level. Social participation in health action becomes a reality at the local level and, at times, it is there that intersectoral action most effectively engages the material and social factors that shape people's health prospects, widening or reducing health equity gaps. One such example is the Health Action Zones in the United Kingdom, which were partner-based entities whose mission was to improve the well-being of disadvantaged groups. Another example is the work of the municipality of Barcelona, in Spain, where a set of interventions, including the reform of primary care, was followed by health improvements in a number of disadvantaged groups, showing that local governments can help reduce health inequities[75].

Local action can also be the starting point for broader structural changes, if it feeds into relevant political decisions and legislation (Box 2.6). Local health services have a critical role to play in this regard, as it is at this level that universal coverage and service delivery reforms meet. Primary care is the way of organizing health-care delivery that is best geared not only to improving health equity, but also to meeting people's other basic needs and expectations.

References

1. Houston S. Matt Anderson's 1939 health plan: how effective and how economical? *Saskatchewan History*, 2005, 57:4–14

2. Xu K et al. Protecting households from catastrophic health spending, *Health Affairs*, 2007, 26:972–983.

3. A conceptual framework for action on the social determinants of health; discussion paper for the Commission on Social Determinants for Health. Geneva, World Health Organization, 2007 (http://www.who.int/social_determinants/resources/csdh_framework_action_05_07.pdf, accessed 19 July 2008)

4. Whitehead M, Dahlgren G. *Concepts and principles for tackling social inequities in health: levelling up part 1.* Copenhagen, World Health Organization Regional Office for Europe, 2006 (Studies on Social and Economic Determinants of Population Health No. 2; http://www.euro.who.int/document/e89383.pdf, accessed 15 July 2008).

5. Adler N, Stewart J. *Reaching for a healthier life. Facts on socioeconomic status and health in the US.* Chicago, JD and CT MacArthur Foundation Research Network on Socioeconomic Status and Health, 2007.

6. Dans A et al. Assessing equity in clinical practice guidelines. *Journal of Clinical Epidemiology*, 2007, 60:540–546.

7. Hart JT. The inverse care law. *Lancet*, 1971, 1:405–412.

8. Gwatkin DR, Bhuiya A, Victora CG. Making health systems more equitable. *Lancet*, 2004, 364:1273–1280.

9. Gilson L, McIntyre D. Post-apartheid challenges: household access and use of care. *International Journal of Health Services*, 2007, 37:673–691.

10. Hanratty B, Zhang T, Whitehead M. How close have universal health systems come to achieving equity in use of curative services? A systematic review. *International Journal of Health Services*, 2007, 37:89–109.

11. Mackenbach JP et al. Strategies to reduce socioeconomic inequalities in health. In: Mackenbach JP, Bakker M, eds. *Reducing inequalities in health: a European perspective.* London, Routledge, 2002.

12. *Report No. 20 (2006-2007): National strategy to reduce social inequalities in health. Paper presented to the Storting.* Oslo, Norwegian Ministry of Health and Care Services, 2007 (http://www.regjeringen.no/en/dep/hod/Documents/regpubl/stmeld/2006-2007/Report-No-20-2006-2007-to-the-Storting.html?id=466505, accessed 19 July 2008).

13. Diderichsen F, Hallqvist J. Social inequalities in health: some methodological considerations for the study of social position and social context. In: Arve-Parès B, ed. *Inequality in health – a Swedish perspective.* Stockholm, Swedish Council for Social Research, 1998.

14. International Labour Office, Deutsche Gesellschaft für Technische Zusammenarbeit (GTZ) Gmbh and World Health Organization. *Extending social protection in health: developing countries, experiences, lessons learnt and recommendations. International Conference on Social Health Insurance in Developing Countries, Berlin, 5–7 December 2005.* Eschborn, Deutsche Gesellschaft für Technische Zusammenarbeit (GTZ) Gmbh, 2007 (http://www2.gtz.de/dokumente/bib/07-0378.pdf, accessed 19 July 2008).

15. *Achieving universal health coverage: developing the health financing system.* Geneva, World Health Organization, Department of Health Systems Financing, 2005 (Technical Briefs for Policy Makers No. 1).

16. *The World Health Report 2000 – Health systems: improving performance.* Geneva, World Health Organization, 2000.

17. Busse R, Schlette S, eds. *Focus on prevention, health and aging and health professions.* Gütersloh, Verlag Bertelsmann Stiftung, 2007 (Health Policy Developments 7/8).

18. Carrin G, Waelkens MP, Criel B. Community-based health insurance in developing countries: a study of its contribution to the performance of health financing systems. *Tropical Medicine and International Health*, 2005, 10:799–811.

19. Jacobs B et al. Bridging community-based health insurance and social protection for health care – a step in the direction of universal coverage? *Tropical Medicine and International Health*, 2008, 13:140–143.

20. *Reclaiming the resources for health. A regional analysis of equity in health in East and Southern Africa.* Kampala, Regional Network on Equity in Health in Southern Africa (EQUINET), 2007.

21. Gilson L. The lessons of user fee experience in Africa. *Health Policy and Planning*, 1997, 12:273–285.

22. Ke X et al. *The elimination of user fees in Uganda: impact on utilization and catastrophic health expenditures.* Geneva, World Health Organization, Department of Health System Financing, Evidence, Information and Policy Cluster, 2005 (Discussion Paper No. 4).

23. Hutton G. *Charting the path to the World Bank's "No blanket policy on user fees". A look over the past 25 years at the shifting support for user fees in health and education, and reflections on the future.* London, Department for International Development (DFID) Health Resource Systems Resource Centre, 2004 (http:www.dfidhealthrc.org/publications/health_sector_financing/04hut01.pdf, accessed 19 July 2008).

24. Tarimo E. *Essential health service packages: uses, abuse and future directions. Current concerns.* Geneva, World Health Organization, 1997 (ARA Paper No. 15; WHO/ARA/CC/97.7).

25. Republica de Chile. *Ley 19.966. Projecto de ley: título I del régimen general de garantías en salud.* Santiago, Ministerio de Salud, 2008 (http://webhosting.redsalud.gov.cl/minsal/archivos/guiasges/leyauge.pdf accessed 19 July 2008).

26. Moccero D. *Delivering cost-efficient public services in health care, education and housing in Chile.* Paris, Organisation for Economic Co-operation and Development, 2008 (Economics Department Working Papers No. 606).

27. Gwatkin DR et al. *Socio-economic differences in health, nutrition, and population within developing countries. An overview.* Washington DC, The World Bank, Human Development Network, Health, Population and Nutrition, and Population Family, 2007 (POPLINE Document Number: 324740).

28. Conway MD, Gupta S, Khajavi K. Addressing Africa's health workforce crisis. *The Mckinsey Quarterly*, November 2007.

29. Bossyns P, Van Lerberghe W. The weakest link: competence and prestige as constraints to referral by isolated nurses in rural Niger. *Human Resources for Health*, 2004, 2:1.

30. Maiga Z, Traoré Nafo F, El Abassi A. La Réforme du secteur santé au Mali, 1989-1996. *Studies in Health Services Organisation & Policy*, 1999, 12:1–132.

31. Abolhassani F. *Primary health care in the Islamic Republic of Iran.* Teheran, Teheran University of Medical Sciences, Health Network Development Centre (unpublished).

32. Naghavi M. *Demographic and health surveys in Iran*, 2008 (personal communication).

33. Porignon D et al. How robust are district health systems? Coping with crisis and disasters in Rutshuru, Democratic Republic of Congo. *Tropical Medicine and International Health*, 1998, 3:559–565.

34. Gauden GI, Powis B, Tamplin SA. Healthy Islands in the Western Pacific – international settings development. *Health Promotion International*, 2000, 15:169–178.

35. *The World Health Report 2006: Working together for health.* Geneva, World Health Organization, 2006.

36. Bossyns P et al. Unaffordable or cost-effective? Introducing an emergency referral system in rural Niger. *Tropical Medicine & International Health*, 2005, 10:879–887.

37. Tibandebage P, Mackintosh M. The market shaping of charges, trust and abuse: health care transactions in Tanzania. *Social Science and Medicine*, 2005, 61:1385–1395.

38. Segall, M et al. *Health care seeking by the poor in transitional economies: the case of Vietnam.* Brighton, Institute of Development Studies, 2000 (IDS Research Reports No. 43).

39. Baru RV. *Private health care in India: social characteristics and trends.* New Delhi, Sage Publications, 1998.

40. Tu NTH, Huong NTL, Diep NB. *Globalisation and its effects on health care and occupational health in Viet Nam.* Geneva, United Nations Research Institute for Social Development, 2003 (http://www.unrisd.org, accessed 19 July 2008).

41. Narayana K. The role of the state in the privatisation and corporatisation of medical care in Andhra Pradesh, India. In: Sen K, ed. *Restructuring health services: changing contexts and comparative perspectives.* London and New Jersey, Zed Books, 2003.

42. Bennett S, McPake B, Mills A. The public/private mix debate in health care. In: Bennett S, McPake B, Mills A, eds. *Private health providers in developing countries. Serving the public interest?* London and New Jersey, Zed Books, 1997.

43. Ogunbekun I, Ogunbekun A, Orobaton N. Private health care in Nigeria: walking the tightrope. *Health Policy and Planning*, 1999, 14:174–181.

44. Mills A, Bennett S, Russell S. *The challenge of health sector reform: what must governments do?* Basingstoke, Palgrave Macmillan, 2001.

45. *The unbearable cost of illness: poverty, ill health and access to healthcare - evidence from Lindi Rural District, Tanzania*, London, Save the Children, 2001.

46. Ferrinho P, Bugalho AM, Van Lerberghe W. Is there a case for privatising reproductive health? Patchy evidence and much wishful thinking. *Studies in Health Services Organisation & Policy*, 2001, 17:343–370.

47. Pan American Health Organization and Swedish International Development Agency. *Exclusion in health in Latin America and the Caribbean.* Washington DC, Pan American Health Organization, 2003 (Extension of Social Protection in Health Series No. 1).

48. Jaffré Y, Olivier de Sardan J-P, eds. *Une médecine inhospitalière. Les difficiles relations entre soignants et soignés dans cinq capitales d'Afrique de l'Ouest*. Paris, Karthala, 2003.

49. Schellenberg JA et al. *Inequalities among the very poor: health care for children in rural southern Tanzania*. Ifakara, Ifakara Health Research and Development Centre, 2002.

50. Oliver A, ed. *Health care priority setting: implications for health inequalities. Proceedings from a meeting of the Health Equity Network*. London, The Nuffield Trust, 2003.

51. *Overcoming obstacles to health: report from the Robert Wood Johnson Foundation to the Commission to Build a Healthier America*. Princeton NJ, Robert Wood Johnson Foundation, 2008.

52. Franks A. *Self-determination background paper. Aboriginal health promotion project*. Lismore NSW, Northern Rivers Area Health Service, Division of Population Health, Health Promotion Unit, 2001 (http://www.ncahs.nsw.gov.au/docs/echidna/ABpaper.pdf, accessed 19 July 2008).

53. *Gathering strength – Canada's Aboriginal action plan: a progress report*. Ottawa, Ministry of Indian Affairs and Northern Development, 2000.

54. King A, Turia T. *He korowai orange – Maori Health Strategy*. Wellington, Ministry of Health of New Zealand, 2002.

55. Cecile MT et al. Gender perspectives and quality of care: towards appropriate and adequate health care for women. *Social Science & Medicine*, 1996, 43:707–720.

56. Murray C, Kulkarni S, Ezzati M. Eight Americas: new perspectives on U.S. health disparities. *American Journal of Preventive Medicine*, 2005, 29:4–10.

57. Paterson I, Judge K. Equality of access to healthcare. In: Mackenbach JP, Bakker M, eds. *Reducing inequalities in health: a European perspective*. London, Routledge, 2002.

58. Doblin L, Leake BD. Ambulatory health services provided to low-income and homeless adult patients in a major community health center. *Journal of General Internal Medicine*, 1996 11:156–162.

59. Frenz P. *Innovative practices for intersectoral action on health: a case study of four programs for social equity. Chilean case study prepared for the CSDH*. Santiago, Ministry of Health, Division of Health Planning, Social Determinants of Health Initiative, 2007.

60. Emanuel EJ, Fuchs VR. Health care vouchers – a proposal for universal coverage. *New England Journal of Medicine*, 2005, 352:1255–1260.

61. Morris S et al. Monetary incentives in primary health care and effects on use and coverage of preventive health care interventions in rural Honduras: cluster randomised trial. *Lancet*, 2004, 364:2030–2037.

62. Armstrong JRM et al. KINET: a social marketing programme of treated nets and net treatment for malaria control in Tanzania, with evaluation of child health and long-term survival. *Transactions of the Royal Society of Tropical Medicine and Hygiene*, 1999, 93:225–231.

63. Adiel K et al. Targeted subsidy for malaria control with treated nets using a discount voucher system in Tanzania. *Health Policy and Planning*, 2003, 18:163–171.

64. Kirby D, Waszak C, Ziegler J. Six school-based clinics: their reproductive health services and impact on sexual behavior. *Family Planning Perspectives*, 1991, 23:6–16.

65. Meng H et al. Effect of a consumer-directed voucher and a disease-management-health-promotion nurse intervention on home care use. *The Gerontologist*, 2005, 45:167–176.

66. Lagarde M, Haines A, Palmer N. Conditional cash transfers for improving uptake of health interventions in low- and middle-income countries. A systematic review. *Journal of the American Medical Association*, 2007, 298:1900–1910.

67. Gwatkin DR, Wagstaff A, Yazbeck A, eds. *Reaching the poor with health, nutrition and population services. What works, what doesn't and why*. Washington DC, The World Bank, 2005.

68. Sretzer, S. The importance of social intervention in Britain's mortality decline, c.1850–1914: a reinterpretation of the role of public health. *Society for the Social History of Medicine*, 1988, 1:1–41.

69. Gwatkin DR. 10 best resources on ... health equity. *Health Policy and Planning*, 2007, 22:348–351.

70. Burström B. Increasing inequalities in health care utilisation across income groups in Sweden during the 1990s? *Health Policy*, 2002, 62:117–129.

71. Whitehead M et al. As the health divide widens in Sweden and Britain, what's happening to access to care? *British Medical Journal*, 1997, 315:1006–1009.

72. Nolen LB et al. Strengthening health information systems to address health equity challenges, *Bulletin of the World Health Organization*, 2005, 83:597–603.

73. Whitehead M, Dahlgren G, Evans T. Equity and health sector reforms: can low-income countries escape the medical poverty trap. *Lancet*, 2001, 358:833–836.

74. Burke MA, Eichler M. The BIAS FREE framework: a practical tool for identifying and eliminating social biases in health research. Geneva, Global Forum for Health Research, 2006 (http://www.globalforumhealth.org/Site/002__What%20we%20do/005__Publications/010__BIAS%20FREE.php, accessed 19 July 2008).

75. Benach J, Borell C, Daponte A. Spain. In: Mackenbach JP, Bakker M, eds. Reducing inequalities in health: a European perspective. London, Routledge, 2002.

76. Balthazar T, Versnick G. *Lokaal sociaal beleidsplan, Gent. Strategisch meerjarenplan 2008-2013*. Gent, Lokaal Sociaal Beleid, 2008 (http://www.lokaalsociaalbeleidgent.be/documenten/publicaties%20LSB-Gent/LSB-plan%20Gent.pdf, accessed 23 July 2008).

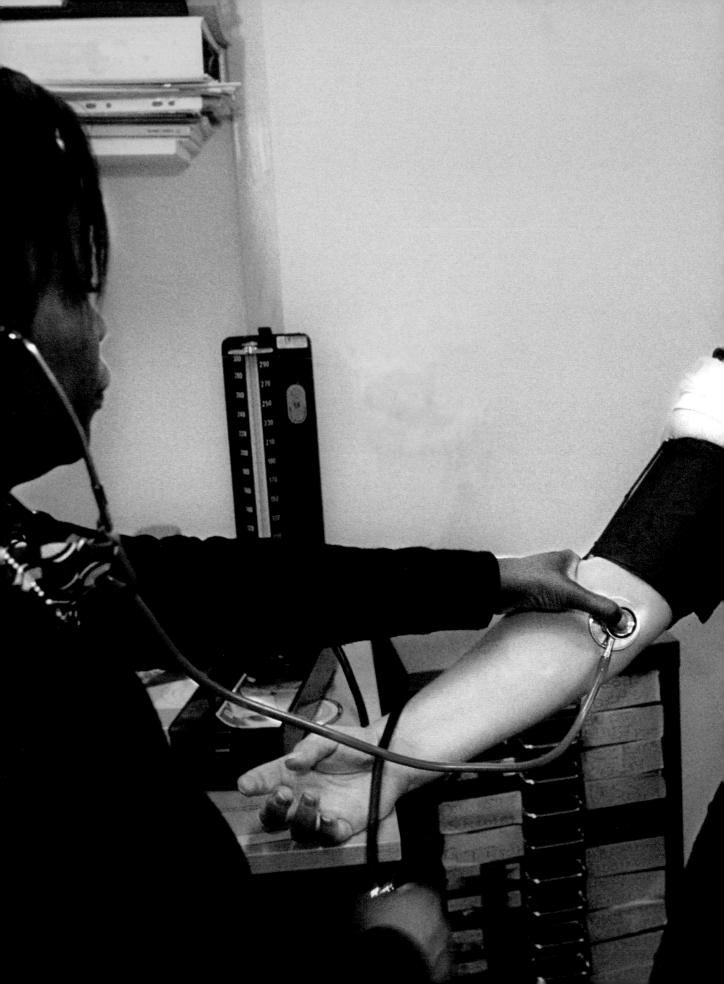

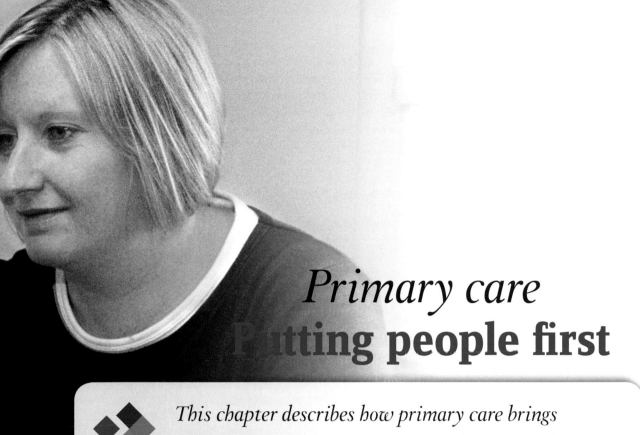

Primary care
Putting people first

This chapter describes how primary care brings promotion and prevention, cure and care together in a safe, effective and socially productive way at the interface between the population and the health system. In short, what needs to be done to achieve this is "to put people first": to give balanced consideration to health and well-being as well as to the values and capacities of the population and the health workers[1]. The chapter starts by describing features of health care that, along with effectiveness and safety, are essential in ensuring improved health and social outcomes.

These features are person-centredness, comprehensiveness and integration, and continuity of care, with a regular point of entry into the health system, so that it becomes possible to build an enduring relationship of trust between people and their health-care providers. The chapter then defines what this implies for the organization of health-care delivery: the necessary switch from specialized to generalist ambulatory care, with responsibility for a defined population and the ability to coordinate support from hospitals, specialized services and civil society organizations.

Good care is about people

Biomedical science is, and should be, at the heart of modern medicine. Yet, as William Osler, one of its founders, pointed out, "it is much more important to know what sort of patient has a disease than what sort of disease a patient has"[2]. Insufficient recognition of the human dimension in health and of the need to tailor the health service's response to the specificity of each community and individual situation represent major shortcomings in contemporary health care, resulting not only in inequity and poor social outcomes, but also diminishing the health outcome returns on the investment in health services.

Putting people first, the focus of service delivery reforms is not a trivial principle. It can require significant – even if often simple – departures from business as usual. The reorganization of a medical centre in Alaska in the United States, accommodating 45 000 patient contacts per year, illustrates how far-reaching the effects can be. The centre functioned to no great satisfaction of either staff or clients until it decided to establish a direct relationship between each individual and family in the community and a specific staff member[3]. The staff were then in a position to know "their" patients' medical history and understand their personal and family situation. People were in a position to get to know and trust their health-care provider: they no longer had to deal with an institution but with their personal caregiver. Complaints about compartmentalized and fragmented services abated[4]. Emergency room visits were reduced by approximately 50% and referrals to specialty care by 30%; waiting times

shortened significantly. With fewer "rebound" visits for unresolved health problems, the workload actually decreased and staff job satisfaction improved. Most importantly, people felt that they were being listened to and respected – a key aspect of what people value about health care[5,6]. A slow bureaucratic system was thus transformed into one that is customer-responsive, customer-owned and customer-driven[4].

In a very different setting, the health centres of Ouallam, a rural district in Niger, implemented an equally straightforward reorganization of their way of working in order to put people first. Rather than the traditional morning curative care consultation and specialized afternoon clinics (growth monitoring, family planning, etc.), the full range of services was offered at all times, while the nurses were instructed to engage in an active dialogue with their patients. For example, they no longer waited for women to ask for contraceptives, but informed them, at every contact, about the range of services available. Within a few months, the very low uptake of family planning, previously attributed to cultural constraints, was a thing of the past (Figure 3.1)[7].

People's experiences of care provided by the health system are determined first and foremost by the way they are treated when they experience a problem and look for help: by the responsiveness of the health-worker interface between population

Figure 3.1 The effect on uptake of contraception of the reorganization of work schedules of rural health centres in Niger

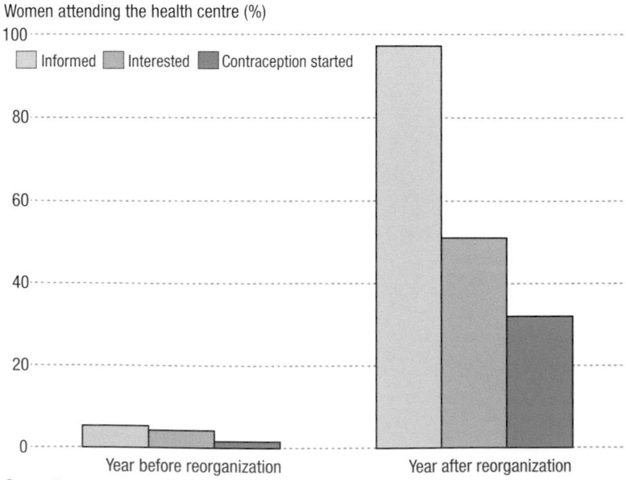

Women attending the health centre (%)

Legend: Informed, Interested, Contraception started

Source: 7

and health services. People value some freedom in choosing a health provider because they want one they can trust and who will attend to them promptly and in an adequate environment, with respect and confidentiality[8].

Health-care delivery can be made more effective by making it more considerate and convenient, as in Ouallam district. However, primary care is about more than shortening waiting times, adapting opening hours or getting staff to be more polite. Health workers have to care for people throughout the course of their lives, as individuals and as members of a family and a community whose health must be protected and enhanced[9], and not merely as body parts with symptoms or disorders that require treating[10].

The service delivery reforms advocated by the PHC movement aim to put people at the centre of health care, so as to make services more effective, efficient and equitable. Health services that do this start from a close and direct relationship between individuals and communities and their caregivers. This, then, provides the basis for person-centredness, continuity, comprehensiveness and integration, which constitute the distinctive features of primary care. Table 3.1 summarizes the differences between primary care and care provided in conventional settings, such as in clinics or hospital outpatient departments, or through the disease control programmes that shape many health services in resource-limited settings. The section that follows reviews these defining features of primary care, and describes how they contribute to better health and social outcomes.

The distinctive features of primary care

Effectiveness and safety are not just technical matters

Health care should be effective and safe. Professionals as well as the general public often over-rate the performance of their health services. The emergence of evidence-based medicine in the 1980s has helped to bring the power and discipline of scientific evidence to health-care decision-making[11], while still taking into consideration patient values and preferences[12]. Over the last decade, several hundred reviews of

Table 3.1 Aspects of care that distinguish conventional health care from people-centred primary care

Conventional ambulatory medical care in clinics or outpatient departments	Disease control programmes	People-centred primary care
Focus on illness and cure	Focus on priority diseases	Focus on health needs
Relationship limited to the moment of consultation	Relationship limited to programme implementation	Enduring personal relationship
Episodic curative care	Programme-defined disease control interventions	Comprehensive, continuous and person-centred care
Responsibility limited to effective and safe advice to the patient at the moment of consultation	Responsibility for disease-control targets among the target population	Responsibility for the health of all in the community along the life cycle; responsibility for tackling determinants of ill-health
Users are consumers of the care they purchase	Population groups are targets of disease-control interventions	People are partners in managing their own health and that of their community

effectiveness have been conducted[13], which have led to better information on the choices available to health practitioners when caring for their patients.

Evidence-based medicine, however, cannot in itself ensure that health care is effective and safe. Growing awareness of the multiple ways in which care may be compromised is contributing to a gradual rise in standards of quality and safety (Box 3.1). Thus far, however, such efforts have concentrated disproportionately on hospital and specialist care, mainly in high- and middle-income countries. The effectiveness and safety of generalist ambulatory care, where most interactions between people and health services take place, has been given much less attention[14]. This is a particularly important issue in the unregulated commercial settings of many developing countries where people often get poor value for money (Box 3.2)[15].

Technical and safety parameters are not the only determinants of the outcomes of health care. The disappointingly low success rate in preventing mother-to-child transmission (MTCT) of HIV in a study in the Côte d'Ivoire (Figure 3.2) illustrates that other features of the organization of health care are equally critical – good drugs are

---

Box 3.1 Towards a science and culture of improvement: evidence to promote patient safety and better outcomes

The outcome of health care results from the balance between the added value of treatment or intervention, and the harm it causes to the patient[16]. Until recently, the extent of such harm has been underestimated. In industrialized countries, approximately 1 in 10 patients suffers harm caused by avoidable adverse events while receiving care[17]: up to 98 000 deaths per year are caused by such events in the United States alone[18]. Multiple factors contribute to this situation[19], ranging from systemic faults to problems of competence, social pressure on patients to undergo risky procedures, to incorrect technology usage[20]. For example, almost 40% of the 16 billion injections administered worldwide each year are given with syringes and needles that are reused without sterilization[14]. Each year, unsafe injections thus cause 1.3 million deaths and almost 26 million years of life lost, mainly because of transmission of hepatitis B and C, and HIV[21].

Especially disquieting is the paucity of information on the extent and determinants of unsafe care in low- and middle-income countries. With unregulated commercialization of care, weaker quality control and health resource limitations, health-care users in low-income countries may well be even more exposed to the risk of unintended patient harm than patients in high-income countries. The World Alliance for Patient Safety[22], among others, advocates making patients safer through systemic interventions and a change in organizational culture rather than through the denunciation of individual health-care practitioners or administrators[23].

Box 3.2 When supplier-induced and consumer-driven demand determine medical advice: ambulatory care in India

"Ms. S is a typical patient who lives in urban Delhi. There are over 70 private-sector medical care providers within a 15-minute walk from her house (and virtually any household in her city). She chooses the private clinic run by Dr. SM and his wife. Above the clinic a prominent sign says "Ms. MM, Gold Medalist, MBBS", suggesting that the clinic is staffed by a highly proficient doctor (an MBBS is the basic degree for a medical doctor as in the British 2 system). As it turns out, Ms. MM is rarely at the clinic. We were told that she sometimes comes at 4 a.m. to avoid the long lines that form if people know she is there. We later discover that she has "franchised" her name to a number of different clinics. Therefore, Ms. S sees Dr. SM and his wife, both of whom were trained in traditional Ayurvedic medicine through a six-month long-distance course. The doctor and his wife sit at a small table surrounded, on one side, by a large number of bottles full of pills, and on the other, a bench with patients on them, which extends into the street. Ms. S sits at the end of this bench. Dr. SM and his wife are the most popular medical care providers in the neighbourhood, with more than 200 patients every day. The doctor spends an average of 3.5 minutes with each patient, asks 3.2 questions, and performs an average of 2.5 examinations. Following the diagnosis, the doctor takes two or three different pills, crushes them using a mortar and pestle, and makes small paper packets from the resulting powder which he gives to Ms. S and asks her to take for two or three days. These medicines usually include one antibiotic and one analgesic and anti-inflammatory drug. Dr. SM tells us that he constantly faces unrealistic patient expectations, both because of the high volume of patients and their demands for treatments that even Dr. SM knows are inappropriate. Dr. SM and his wife seem highly motivated to provide care to their patients and even with a very crowded consultation room they spend more time with their patients than a public sector doctor would. However, they are not bound by their knowledge [...] and instead deliver health care like the crushed pills in a paper packet, which will result in more patients willing to pay more for their services"[24].

not enough. How services deal with people is also vitally important. Surveys in Australia, Canada, Germany, New Zealand, the United Kingdom and the United States show that a high number of patients report safety risks, poor care coordination and deficiencies in care for chronic conditions[25]. Communication is often inadequate and lacking in information on treatment schedules. Nearly one in every two patients feels that doctors only rarely or never asked their opinion about treatment. Patients may consult different providers for related or even for the same conditions which, given the lack of coordination among these providers, results in duplication and contradictions[25]. This situation is similar to that reported in other countries, such as Ethiopia[26], Pakistan[27] and Zimbabwe[28].

There has, however, been progress in recent years. In high-income countries, confrontation with chronic disease, mental health problems, multi-morbidity and the social dimension of disease has focused attention on the need for more comprehensive and person-centred approaches and continuity of care. This resulted not only from client pressure, but also from professionals who realized the critical importance of such

Figure 3.2 Lost opportunities for prevention of mother-to-child transmission of HIV (MTCT) in Côte d'Ivoire[29]: only a tiny fraction of the expected transmissions are actually prevented

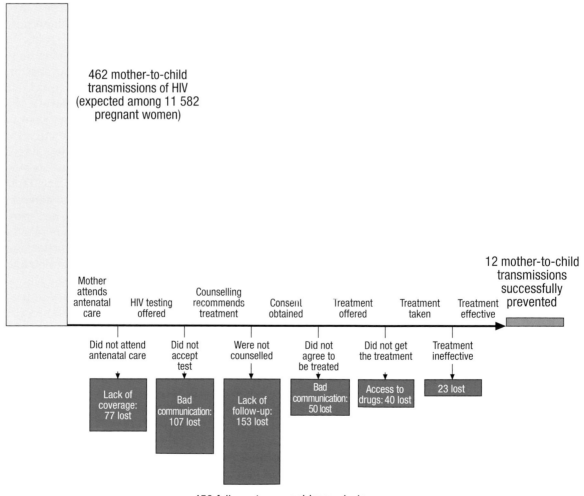

features of care in achieving better outcomes for their patients. Many health professionals have begun to appreciate the limitations of narrow clinical approaches, for example, to cardiovascular disease. As a result there has been a welcome blurring of the traditional boundaries between curative care, preventive medicine and health promotion.

In low-income countries, this evolution is also visible. In recent years, many of the programmes targeting infectious disease priorities have given careful consideration to comprehensiveness, continuity and patient-centredness. Maternal and child health services have often been at the forefront of these attempts, organizing a continuum of care and a comprehensive approach. This process has been consolidated through the joint UNICEF/WHO Integrated Management of Childhood Illness initiatives[30]. Their experience with programmes such as the WHO's Extended Programme for Immunization has put health professionals in many developing countries a step ahead compared to their high-income country colleagues, as they more readily see themselves responsible not just for patients, but also for population coverage. More recently, HIV/AIDS programmes have drawn the attention of providers and policy-makers to the importance of counselling, continuity of care, the complementarity of prevention, treatment and palliation and critically, to the value of empathy and listening to patients.

Understanding people: person-centred care

When people are sick they are a great deal less concerned about managerial considerations of productivity, health targets, cost-effectiveness and rational organization than about their own predicament. Each individual has his or her own way of experiencing and coping with health problems within their specific life circumstances[31]. Health workers have to be able to handle that diversity. For health workers at the interface between the population and the health services, the challenge is much more complicated than for a specialized referral service: managing a well-defined disease is a relatively straightforward technical challenge. Dealing with health problems, however, is complicated as people need to

be understood holistically: their physical, emotional and social concerns, their past and their future, and the realities of the world in which they live. Failure to deal with the whole person in their specific familial and community contexts misses out on important aspects of health that do not immediately fit into disease categories. Partner violence against women (Box 3.3), for example, can be detected, prevented or mitigated by health services that are sufficiently close to the communities they serve and by health workers who know the people in their community.

People want to know that their health worker understands them, their suffering and the constraints they face. Unfortunately, many providers neglect this aspect of the therapeutic relation, particularly when they are dealing with disadvantaged groups. In many health services, responsiveness and person-centredness are treated as luxury goods to be handed out only to a selected few.

Over the last 30 years, a considerable body of research evidence has shown that person-centredness is not only important to relieve the patient's anxiety but also to improve the provider's job satisfaction[50]. The response to a health problem is more likely to be effective if the provider understands its various dimensions[51]. For a start, simply asking patients how they feel about their illness, how it affects their lives, rather than focusing only on the disease, results in measurably increased trust and compliance[52] that allows patient and provider to find a common ground on clinical management, and facilitates the integration of prevention and health promotion in the therapeutic response[50,51]. Thus, person-centredness becomes the "clinical method of participatory democracy"[53], measurably improving the quality of care, the success of treatment and the quality of life of those benefiting from such care (Table 3.2).

In practice, clinicians rarely address their patients' concerns, beliefs and understanding of illness, and seldom share problem management options with them[58]. They limit themselves to simple technical prescriptions, ignoring the complex human dimensions that are critical to the appropriateness and effectiveness of the care they provide[59].

Box 3.3 The health-care response to partner violence against women

Intimate partner violence has numerous well-documented consequences for women's health (and for the health of their children), including injuries, chronic pain syndromes, unintended and unwanted pregnancies, pregnancy complications, sexually transmitted infections and a wide range of mental health problems[32,33,34,35,36,37]. Women suffering from violence are frequent health-care users [38,39].

Health workers are, therefore, well placed to identify and provide care to the victims of violence, including referral for psychosocial, legal and other support. Their interventions can reduce the impact of violence on a woman's health and well-being, and that of her children, and can also help prevent further violence.

Research has shown that most women think health-care providers should ask about violence[40]. While they do not expect them to solve their problem, they would like to be listened to and treated in a non-judgemental way and get the support they need to take control over their decisions. Health-care providers often find it difficult to ask women about violence. They lack the time and the training and skills to do it properly, and are reluctant to be involved in judicial proceedings.

The most effective approach for health providers to use when responding to violence is still a matter of debate[41]. They are generally advised to ask all women about intimate partner abuse as a routine part of any health assessment, usually referred to as "screening" or routine enquiry[42]. Several reviews found that this technique increased the rate of identification of women experiencing violence in antenatal and primary-care clinics, but there was little evidence that this was sustained[40], or was effective in terms of health outcomes[43]. Among women who have stayed in shelters, there is evidence that those who received a specific counselling and advocacy service reported a lower rate of re-abuse and an improved quality of life[44]. Similarly, among women experiencing violence during pregnancy, those who received "empowerment counselling" reported improved functioning and less psychological and non-severe physical abuse, and had lower postnatal depression scores[45].

While there is still no consensus on the most effective strategy, there is growing agreement that health services should aim to identify and support women experiencing violence[46], and that health-care providers should be well educated about these issues, as they are essential in building capacity and skills. Health-care providers should, as a minimum, be informed about violence against women, its prevalence and impact on health, when to suspect it and how to best respond. Clearly, there are technical dimensions to this. For example, in the case of sexual assault, providers need to be able to provide the necessary treatment and care, including provision of emergency contraception and prophylaxis for sexually transmitted infections, including HIV where relevant, as well as psychosocial support. There are other dimensions too: health workers need to be able to document any injuries as completely and carefully as possible[47,48,49] and they need to know how to work with communities – in particular with men and boys – on changing attitudes and practices related to gender inequality and violence.

Table 3.2 Person-centredness: evidence of its contribution to quality of care and better outcomes

Improved treatment intensity and quality of life – Ferrer (2005)[54]
Better understanding of the psychological aspects of a patient's problems – Gulbrandsen (1997)[55]
Improved satisfaction with communication – Jaturapatporn (2007)[56]
Improved patient confidence regarding sensitive problems – Kovess-Masféty (2007)[57]
Increased trust and treatment compliance – Fiscella (2004)[52]
Better integration of preventive and promotive care – Mead (1982)[50]

Thus, technical advice on lifestyle, treatment schedule or referral all too often neglects not only the constraints of the environment in which people live, but also their potential for self-help in dealing with a host of health problems ranging from diarrhoeal disease[60] to diabetes management[61]. Yet, neither the nurse in Niger's rural health centre nor the general practitioner in Belgium can, for example, refer a patient to hospital without negotiating[62,63]: along with medical criteria, they have to take into account the patient's values, the family's values, and their lifestyle and life perspective[64].

Few health providers have been trained for person-centred care. Lack of proper preparation is compounded by cross-cultural conflicts, social stratification, discrimination and stigma[63]. As a consequence, the considerable potential of people to contribute to their own health through lifestyle, behaviour and self-care, and by adapting

---

Box 3.4 Empowering users to contribute to their own health

Families can be empowered to make choices that are relevant to their health. Birth and emergency plans[66], for example, are based on a joint examination between the expectant mother and health staff – well before the birth – of her expectations regarding childbirth. Issues discussed include where the birth will take place, and how support for care of the home and any other children will be organized while the woman is giving birth. The discussion can cover planning for expenses, arrangements for transport and medical supplies, as well as identification of a compatible blood donor in case of haemorrhage. Such birth plans are being implemented in countries as diverse as Egypt, Guatemala, Indonesia, the Netherlands and the United Republic of Tanzania. They constitute one example of how people can participate in decisions relating to their health in a way that empowers them[67]. Empowerment strategies can improve health and social outcomes through several pathways; the condition for success is that they are embedded in local contexts and based on a strong and direct relationship between people and their health workers[68]. The strategies can relate to a variety of areas, as shown below:

- developing household capacities to stay healthy, make healthy decisions and respond to emergencies – France's self-help organization of diabetics[69], South Africa's family empowerment and parent training programmes[70], the United Republic of Tanzania's negotiated treatment plans for safe motherhood[71], and Mexico's active ageing programme[72];
- increasing citizens' awareness of their rights, needs and potential problems – Chile's information on entitlements[73] and Thailand's Declaration of Patients' Rights[74];
- strengthening linkages for social support within communities and with the health system – support and advice to family caregivers dealing with dementia in developing country settings[75], Bangladesh's rural credit programmes and their impact on care-seeking behaviour[76], and Lebanon's neighbourhood environment initiatives[77].

---

professional advice optimally to their life circumstances is underutilized. There are numerous, albeit often missed, opportunities to empower people to participate in decisions that affect their own health and that of their families (Box 3.4). They require health-care providers who can relate to people and assist them in making informed choices. The current payment systems and incentives in community health-care delivery often work against establishing this type of dialogue[65]. Conflicts of interest between provider and patient, particularly in unregulated commercial settings, are a major disincentive to person-centred care. Commercial providers may be more courteous and client-friendly than in the average health centre, but this is no substitute for person-centredness.

Comprehensive and integrated responses

The diversity of health needs and challenges that people face does not fit neatly into the discrete diagnostic categories of textbook promotive, preventive, curative or rehabilitative care[78,79]. They call for the mobilization of a comprehensive range of resources that may include health promotion and prevention interventions as well as diagnosis and treatment or referral, chronic or long-term home care, and, in some models, social services[80]. It is at the entry point of the system, where people

first present their problem, that the need for a comprehensive and integrated offer of care is most critical.

Comprehensiveness makes managerial and operational sense and adds value (Table 3.3). People take up services more readily if they know a comprehensive spectrum of care is on offer. Moreover, it maximizes opportunities for preventive care and health promotion while reducing unnecessary reliance on specialized or hospital care[81]. Specialization has its comforts, but the fragmentation it induces is often visibly counterproductive and inefficient: it makes no sense to monitor the growth of children and neglect the health of their mothers (and vice versa), or to treat someone's tuberculosis without considering their HIV status or whether they smoke.

Table 3.3 Comprehensiveness: evidence of its contribution to quality of care and better outcomes

Better health outcomes – Forrest (1996)[82], Chande (1996)[83], Starfield (1998)[84]
Increased uptake of disease-focused preventive care (e.g. blood pressure screen, mammograms, pap smears) – Bindman (1996)[85]
Fewer patients admitted for preventable complications of chronic conditions – Shea (1992)[86]

That does not mean that entry-point health workers should solve all the health problems that are presented there, nor that all health programmes always need to be delivered through a single integrated service-delivery point. Nevertheless, the primary-care team has to be able to respond to the bulk of health problems in the community. When it cannot do so, it has to be able to mobilize other resources, by referring or by calling for support from specialists, hospitals, specialized diagnostic and treatment centres, public-health programmes, long-term care services, home-care or social services, or self-help and other community organizations. This cannot mean giving up responsibility: the primary-care team remains responsible for helping people to navigate this complex environment.

Comprehensive and integrated care for the bulk of the assorted health problems in the community is more efficient than relying on separate services for selected problems, partly because it leads to a better knowledge of the population and builds greater trust. One activity reinforces the other. Health services that offer a comprehensive range of services increase the uptake and coverage of, for example, preventive programmes, such as cancer screening or vaccination (Figure 3.3). They prevent complications and improve health outcomes.

Comprehesive services also facilitate early detection and prevention of problems, even in the absence of explicit demand. There are individuals and groups who could benefit from care even if they express no explicit spontaneous demand, as in the case of women attending the health centres in Ouallam district, Niger, or people with undiagnosed high blood pressure or depression. Early detection of disease, preventive care to reduce the incidence of poor health, health promotion to reduce risky behaviour, and addressing social and other determinants of health all require the health service to take the initiative. For many problems, local health workers are the only ones who are in a position to effectively address problems in the community: they are the only ones, for example, in a position to assist parents with care in early childhood development, itself an important determinant of later health, well-being and productivity[87]. Such interventions require proactive health teams offering a comprehensive

range of services. They depend on a close and trusting relationship between the health services and the communities they serve, and, thus, on health workers who know the people in their community[88].

Continuity of care

Understanding people and the context in which they live is not only important in order to provide a comprehensive, person-centred response, it also conditions continuity of care. Providers often behave as if their responsibility starts when a patient walks in and ends when they leave the premises. Care should not, however, be limited to the moment a patient consults nor be confined to the four walls of the consultation room. Concern for outcomes mandates a consistent and coherent approach to the management of the patient's problem, until the problem is resolved or the risk that justified follow-up has disappeared. Continuity of care is an important determinant of effectiveness, whether for chronic disease management, reproductive health, mental health or for making sure children grow up healthily (Table 3.4).

Figure 3.3 More comprehensive health centres have better vaccination coverage[a,b]

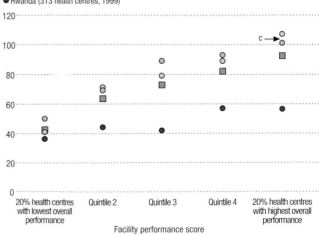

DPT3 vaccination coverage (%)
◉ Democratic Republic of the Congo (380 health centres, 2004)
◎ Madagascar (534 health centres, 2006)
▣ Weighted average of coverage in each country quintile
● Rwanda (313 health centres, 1999)

Facility performance score

[a] Total 1227 health centres, covering a population of 16 million people.
[b] Vaccination coverage was not included in the assessment of overall health-centre performance across a range of services.
[c] Includes vaccination of children not belonging to target population.

Table 3.4 Continuity of care: evidence of its contribution to quality of care and better outcomes

Lower all-cause mortality – Shi (2003)[90], Franks (1998)[91], Villalbi (1999)[92], PAHO (2005)[93]

Better access to care – Weinick (2000)[94], Forrest (1998)[95]

Less re-hospitalization – Weinberger (1996)[96]

Fewer consultations with specialists – Woodward (2004)[97]

Less use of emergency services – Gill (2000)[98]

Better detection of adverse effects of medical interventions – Rothwell (2005)[99], Kravitz (2004)[100]

Continuity of care depends on ensuring continuity of information as people get older, when they move from one residence to another, or when different professionals interact with one particular individual or household. Access to medical records and discharge summaries, electronic, conventional or client-held, improves the choice of the course of treatment and of coordination of care. In Canada, for example, one in seven people attending an emergency department had medical information missing that was very likely to result in patient harm[101]. Missing information is a common cause of delayed care and uptake of unnecessary services[102]. In the United States, it is associated with 15.6% of all reported errors in ambulatory care[103]. Today's information and communication technologies, albeit under-utilized, gives unprecedented possibilities to improve the circulation of medical information at an affordable cost[104], thus enhancing continuity, safety and learning (Box 3.5). Moreover, it is no longer the exclusive privilege of high-resource environments, as the Open Medical Record System demonstrates: electronic health records developed through communities of practice and open-source software are facilitating continuity and quality of care for patients with HIV/AIDS in many low-income countries[105].

Better patient records are necessary but not sufficient. Health services need to make active efforts to minimize the numerous obstacles to continuity of care. Compared to payment by capitation or by fee-for-episode, out-of-pocket fee-for-service payment is a common deterrent, not only to access, but also to continuity of care[107]. In Singapore, for example, patients were formerly not allowed to use their health savings account (Medisave) for outpatient treatment, resulting in patient delays and lack of treatment compliance for the chronically ill. This had become so problematic that regulations were changed. Hospitals are now encouraged to transfer patients with diabetes, high blood pressure, lipid disorder and stroke to registered general practitioners, with Medisave accounts covering ambulatory care[108].

Other barriers to continuity include treatment schedules requiring frequent clinic attendance that carry a heavy cost in time, travel expenses or lost wages. They may be ill-understood and patient motivation may be lacking. Patients may get lost in the complicated institutional environment of referral hospitals or social services. Such problems need to be anticipated and recognized at an early stage. The effort required from health workers is not negligible: negotiating the modalities of the treatment schedule with the patients so as to maximize the chances that it can be completed; keeping registries of clients with chronic conditions; and creating communication channels through home visits, liaison with community workers, telephonic reminders and text messages to re-establish interrupted continuity. These mundane tasks often make the difference between a successful outcome and a treatment failure, but are rarely rewarded. They are much easier to implement when patient and caregiver have clearly identified how and by whom follow-up will be organized.

A regular and trusted provider as entry point

Comprehensiveness, continuity and person-centredness are critical to better health outcomes. They all depend on a stable, long-term, personal relationship (a feature also called "longitudinality"[84]) between the population and the professionals who are their entry point to the health system.

Most ambulatory care in conventional settings is not organized to build such relationships. The busy, anonymous and technical environment of hospital outpatient departments, with their many specialists and sub-specialists, produce mechanical interactions between nameless individuals and an institution – not people-centred care. Smaller clinics are less anonymous, but the care they provide is often more akin to a commercial or administrative transaction that starts and ends with the consultation than to a responsive problem-solving exercise. In this regard, private clinics do not perform differently than public health centres[64]. In the rural areas of low-income countries, governmental health centres are usually designed to work in close relationship with the community they serve. The reality is often different. Earmarking of resources and staff for selected programmes is increasingly leading to fragmentation[109], while the lack of funds, the

pauperization of the health staff and rampant commercialization makes building such relationships difficult[110]. There are many examples to the contrary, but the relationship between providers and their clients, particularly the poorer ones, is often not conducive to building relationships of understanding, empathy and trust[62].

Building enduring relationships requires time. Studies indicate that it takes two to five years before its full potential is achieved[84] but, as the Alaska health centre mentioned at the beginning of this chapter shows, it drastically changes the way care is being provided. Access to the same team of health-care providers over time fosters the development of a relationship of trust between the individual and their health-care provider[97,111,112]. Health professionals are more likely to respect and understand patients they know

---

Box 3.5 Using information and communication technologies to improve access, quality and efficiency in primary care

Information and communication technologies enable people in remote and underserved areas to have access to services and expertise otherwise unavailable to them, especially in countries with uneven distribution or chronic shortages of physicians, nurses and health technicians or where access to facilities and expert advice requires travel over long distances. In such contexts, the goal of improved access to health care has stimulated the adoption of technology for remote diagnosis, monitoring and consultation. Experience in Chile of immediate transmission of electrocardiograms in cases of suspected myocardial infarction is a noteworthy example: examination is carried out in an ambulatory setting and the data are sent to a national centre where specialists confirm the diagnosis via fax or e-mail. This technology-facilitated consultation with experts allows rapid response and appropriate treatment where previously it was unavailable. The Internet is a key factor in its success, as is the telephone connectivity that has been made available to all health facilities in the country.

A further benefit of using information and communication technologies in primary-care services is the improved quality of care. Health-care providers are not only striving to deliver more effective care, they are also striving to deliver safer care. Tools, such as electronic health records, computerized prescribing systems and clinical decision aids, support practitioners in providing safer care in a range of settings. For example, in a village in western Kenya, electronic health records integrated with laboratory, drug procurement and reporting systems have drastically reduced clerical labour and errors, and have improved follow-up care.

As the costs of delivering health care continue to rise, information and communication technologies provide new avenues for personalized, citizen-centred and home-centred care. Towards this end, there has been significant investment in research and development of consumer-friendly applications. In Cape Town, South Africa, an "on cue compliance service" takes the names and mobile telephone numbers of patients with tuberculosis (supplied by a clinic) and enters them into a database. Every half an hour, the on cue server reads the database and sends personalized SMS messages to the patients, reminding them to take their medication. The technology is low-cost and robust. Cure and completion rates are similar to those of patients receiving clinic-based DOTS, but at lower cost to both clinic and patient, and in a way that interferes much less with everyday life than the visits to the clinic[106]. In the same concept of supporting lifestyles linked to primary care, network devices have become a key element of an innovative community programme in the Netherlands, where monitoring and communication devices are built into smart apartments for senior citizens. This system reduces clinic visits and facilitates living independently with chronic diseases that require frequent checks and adjustment of medications.

Many clinicians who want to promote health and prevent illness are placing high hopes in the Internet as the place to go for health advice to complement or replace the need to seek the advice of a health professional. New applications, services and access to information have permanently altered the relationships between consumers and health professionals, putting knowledge directly into people's own hands.

Table 3.5 Regular entry point: evidence of its contribution to quality of care and better outcomes

Increased satisfaction with services – Weiss (1996)[116], Rosenblatt (1998)[117], Freeman (1997)[124], Miller (2000)[125]
Better compliance and lower hospitalization rate – Weiss (1996)[116], Rosenblatt (1998)[117], Freeman (1997)[124], Mainous (1998)[126]
Less use of specialists and emergency services – Starfield (1998)[82], Parchman (1994)[127], Hurley (1989)[128], Martin (1989)[129], Gadomski (1998)[130]
Fewer consultations with specialists – Hurley (1989)[128], Martin (1989)[129]
More efficient use of resources – Forrest (1996)[82], Forrest (1998)[95], Hjortdahl (1991)[131], Roos (1998)[132]
Better understanding of the psychological aspects of a patient's problem – Gulbrandsen (1997)[55]
Better uptake of preventive care by adolescents – Ryan (2001)[133]
Protection against over-treatment – Schoen (2007)[134]

well, which creates more positive interaction and better communication[113]. They can more readily understand and anticipate obstacles to continuity of care, follow up on the progress and assess how the experience of illness or disability is affecting the individual's daily life. More mindful of the circumstances in which people live, they can tailor care to the specific needs of the person and recognize health problems at earlier stages.

This is not merely a question of building trust and patient satisfaction, however important these may be[114,115]. It is worthwhile because it leads to better quality and better outcomes (Table 3.5). People who use the same source of care for most of their health-care needs tend to comply better with advice given, rely less on emergency services, require less hospitalization and are more satisfied with care[98 116,117,118]. Providers save consultation time, reduce the use of laboratory tests and costs[95,119,120], and increase uptake of preventive care[121]. Motivation improves through the social recognition built up by such relationships. Still, even dedicated health professionals will not seize all these opportunities spontaneously[122,123].

The interface between the population and their health services needs to be designed in a way that not only makes this possible, but also the most likely course of action.

Organizing primary-care networks

A health service that provides entry point ambulatory care for health- and health-related problems should, thus, offer a comprehensive range of integrated diagnostic, curative, rehabilitative and palliative services. In contrast to most conventional health-care delivery models, the offer of services should include prevention and promotion as well as efforts to tackle determinants of ill-health locally. A direct and enduring relationship between the provider and the people in the community served is essential to be able to take into account the personal and social context of patients and their families, ensuring continuity of care over time as well as across services.

In order for conventional health services to be transformed into primary care, i.e. to ensure that these distinctive features get due prominence, they must reorganized. A precondition is to ensure that they become directly and permanently accessible, without undue reliance on out-of-pocket payments and with social protection offered by universal coverage schemes. But another set of arrangements is critical for the transformation of conventional care – ambulatory- and institution-based, generalist and specialist – into local networks of primary-care centres[135,136,137,138,139,140]:

- bringing care closer to people, in settings in close proximity and direct relationship with the community, relocating the entry point to the health system from hospitals and specialists to close-to-client generalist primary-care centres;
- giving primary-care providers the responsibility for the health of a defined population, in its entirety: the sick and the healthy, those who choose to consult the services and those who choose not to do so;
- strengthening primary-care providers' role as coordinators of the inputs of other levels of care by giving them administrative authority and purchasing power.

Bringing care closer to the people

A first step is to relocate the entry point to the health system from specialized clinics, hospital outpatient departments and emergency services, to generalist ambulatory care in close-to-client settings. Evidence has been accumulating that this transfer carries measurable benefits in terms of relief from suffering, prevention of illness and death, and improved health equity. These findings hold true in both national and cross-national studies, even if all of the distinguishing features of primary care are not fully realized[31].

Generalist ambulatory care is more likely or as likely to identify common life-threatening conditions as specialist care[141,142]. Generalists adhere to clinical practice guidelines to the same extent as specialists[143], although they are slower to adopt them[144,145]. They prescribe fewer invasive interventions[146,147,148,149], fewer and shorter hospitalizations[127,133,119] and have a greater focus on preventive care[133,150]. This results in lower overall health-care costs[82] for similar health outcomes[146,151,152,153,154,155] and greater patient satisfaction[125,150,156]. Evidence from comparisons between high-income countries shows that higher proportions of generalist professionals working in ambulatory settings are associated with lower overall costs and higher quality rankings[157]. Conversely, countries that increase reliance on specialists have stagnating or declining health outcomes when measured at the population level, while fragmentation of care exacerbates user dissatisfaction and contributes to a growing divide between health and social services[157,158,159]. Information on low- and middle-income countries is harder to obtain[160], but there are indications that patterns are similar. Some studies estimate that in Latin America and the Caribbean more reliance on generalist care could avoid one out of two hospital admissions[161]. In Thailand, generalist ambulatory care outside a hospital context has been shown to be more patient-centred and responsive as well as cheaper and less inclined to over-medicalization[162] (Figure 3.4).

The relocation of the entry point into the system from specialist hospital to generalist ambulatory care creates the conditions for more comprehensiveness, continuity and person-centredness. This amplifies the benefits of the relocation. It is particularly the case when services are organized as a dense network of small, close-to-client service delivery points. This makes it easier to have teams that are small enough to know their communities and be known by them, and stable enough to establish an enduring relationship. These teams require relational and organizational capacities as much as the technical competencies to solve the bulk of health problems locally.

Responsibility for a well-identified population

In conventional ambulatory care, the provider assumes responsibility for the person attending the consultation for the duration of the consultation and, in the best of circumstances, that responsibility extends to ensuring continuity of care. This passive, response-to-demand approach fails to help a considerable number of people who could benefit from care. There are people who, for various reasons, are, or feel, excluded from access to services and do not take up care even when they are in need. There are people who suffer illness but delay seeking care. Others present risk factors and could benefit from screening or prevention programmes (e.g. for cervical cancer or for childhood obesity), but are left out because they do not consult: preventive services that are limited to service users often leave out those most in need[163]. A passive, response-to-demand

Figure 3.4 Inappropriate investigations prescribed for simulated patients presenting with a minor stomach complaint, Thailand[a,b,162]

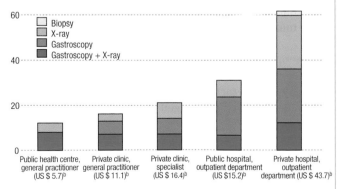

Patients for whom inappropriate investigations were prescribed (%)

a Observation made in 2000, before introduction of Thailand's universal coverage scheme.
b Cost to the patient, including doctor's fees, drugs, laboratory and technical investigations.

approach has a second untoward consequence: it lacks the ambition to deal with local determinants of ill-health – whether social, environmental or work-related. All this represents lost opportunities for generating health: providers that only assume responsibility for their customers concentrate on repairing rather than on maintaining and promoting health.

The alternative is to entrust each primary-care team with the explicit responsibility for a well-defined community or population. They can then be held accountable, through administrative measures or contractual arrangements, for providing comprehensive, continuous and person-centred care to that population, and for mobilizing a comprehensive range of support services – from promotive through to palliative. The simplest way of assigning responsibility is to identify the community served on the basis of geographical criteria – the classic approach in rural areas. The simplicity of geographical assignment, however, is deceptive. It follows an administrative, public sector logic that often has problems adapting to the emergence of a multitude of other providers. Furthermore, administrative geography may not coincide with sociological reality, especially in urban areas. People move around and may work in a different area than where they live, making the health unit closest to home actually an inconvenient source of care. More importantly, people value choice and may resent an administrative assignment to a particular health unit. Some countries find geographical criteria of proximity the most appropriate to define who fits in the population of responsibility, others rely on active registration or patient lists. The important point is not how but whether the population is well identified and mechanisms exist to ensure that nobody is left out.

Once such explicit comprehensive responsibilities for the health of a well-identified and defined population are assigned, with the related financial and administrative accountability mechanisms, the rules change.

■ The primary-care team has to broaden the portfolio of care it offers, developing activities and programmes that can improve outcomes, but which they might otherwise neglect[164]. This sets the stage for investment in prevention and promotion activities, and for venturing into areas that are often overlooked, such as health in schools and in the workplace. It forces the primary-care team to reach out to and work with organizations and individuals within the community: volunteers and community health workers who act as the liaison with patients or animate grassroots community groups, social workers, self-help groups, etc.

■ It forces the team to move out of the four walls of their consultation room and reach out to the people in the community. This can bring significant health benefits. For example, large-scale programmes, based on home-visits and community animation, have been shown to be effective in reducing risk factors for neonatal mortality and actual mortality rates. In the United States, such programmes have reduced neonatal mortality by 60% in some settings[165]. Part of the benefit is due to better uptake of effective care by people who would otherwise remain deprived. In Nepal, for example, the community dynamics of women's groups led to the better uptake of care, with neonatal and maternal mortality lower than in control communities by 29% and 80%, respectively[166].

■ It forces the team to take targeted initiatives, in collaboration with other sectors, to reach the excluded and the unreached and tackle broader determinants of ill-health. As Chapter 2 has shown, this is a necessary complement to establishing universal coverage and one where local health services play a vital role. The 2003 heatwave in western Europe, for example, highlighted the importance of reaching out to the isolated elderly and the dramatic consequences of failing to do so: an excess mortality of more than 50 000 people[167].

For people and communities, formal links with an identifiable source of care enhance the likelihood that long-term relationships will develop; that services are encouraged to pay more attention to the defining features of primary care; and that lines of communication are more intelligible. At the same time, coordination linkages can be formalized with other levels of care – specialists, hospitals or other technical services – and with social services.

The primary-care team as a hub of coordination

Primary-care teams cannot ensure comprehensive responsibility for their population without support from specialized services, organizations and institutions that are based outside the community served. In resource-constrained circumstances, these sources of support will typically be concentrated in a "first referral level district hospital". Indeed, the classic image of a health-care system based on PHC is that of a pyramid with the district hospital at the top and a set of (public) health centres that refer to the higher authority.

In conventional settings, ambulatory care professionals have little say in how hospitals and specialized services contribute – or fail to contribute – to the health of their patients, and feel little inclination to reach out to other institutions and stakeholders that are relevant to the health of the local community. This changes if they are entrusted with responsibility for a defined population and are recognized as the regular point of entry for that population. As health-care networks expand, the health-care landscape becomes far more crowded and pluralistic. More resources allow for diversification: the range of specialized services that comes within reach may include emergency services, specialists, diagnostic infrastructure, dialysis centres, cancer screening, environmental technicians, long-term care institutions, pharmacies, etc. This represents new opportunities, provided the primary-care teams can assist their community in making the best use of that potential, which is particularly critical to public health, mental health and long-term care[168].

The coordination (or gatekeeping) role this entails effectively transforms the primary-care pyramid into a network, where the relations between the primary-care team and the other institutions and services are no longer based only on top-down hierarchy and bottom-up referral, but on cooperation and coordination (Figure 3.5). The primary-care team then becomes the mediator between the community and the other levels

Figure 3.5 Primary care as a hub of coordination: networking within the community served and with outside partners[173,174]

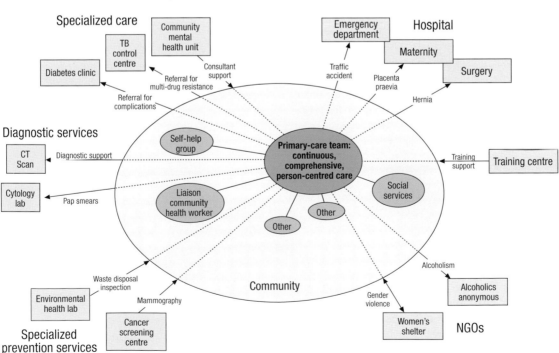

of the health system, helping people navigate the maze of health services and mobilizing the support of other facilities by referring patients or calling on the support of specialized services.

This coordination and mediation role also extends to collaboration with other types of organizations, often nongovernmental. These can provide significant support to local primary care. They can help ensure that people know what they are entitled to and have the information to avoid substandard providers[169,170]. Independent ombudsman structures or consumer organizations can help users handle complaints. Most importantly, there is a wealth of self-help and mutual support associations for diabetics, people living with handicaps and chronic diseases that can help people to help themselves[171]. In the United States alone, more than five million people belong to mutual help groups while, in recent years, civil society organizations dealing with health and health-related issues, from self-help to patient's rights, have been mushrooming in many low- and middle-income countries. These groups do much more than just inform patients. They help people take charge of their own situation, improve their health, cope better with ill-health, increase self-confidence and diminish over-medicalization[172]. Primary-care teams can only be strengthened by reinforcing their linkages with such groups.

Where primary-care teams are in a position to take on this coordinator role, their work becomes more rewarding and attractive, while the overall effects on health are positive. Reliance on specialists and hospitalization is reduced by filtering out unnecessary uptake, whereas patient delay is reduced for those who do need referral care, the duration of their hospitalization is shortened, and post-hospitalization follow-up is improved[83,128,129].

The coordination function provides the institutional framework for mobilizing across sectors to secure the health of local communities. It is not an optional extra but an essential part of the remit of primary-care teams. This has policy implications: coordination will remain wishful thinking unless the primary-care team has some form of either administrative or financial leverage. Coordination also depends on the different institutions'

recognition of the key role of the primary-care teams. Current professional education systems, career structure and remuneration mechanisms most often give signals to the contrary. Reversing these well-entrenched disincentives to primary care requires strong leadership.

Monitoring progress

The switch from conventional to primary care is a complex process that cannot be captured in a single, universal metric. Only in recent years has it been possible to start disentangling the effects of the various features that define primary care. In part, this is because the identification of the features that make the difference between primary care and conventional health-care delivery has taken years of trial and error, and the instruments to measure them have not been generalized. This is because these features are never all put into place as a single package of reforms, but are the result of a gradual shaping and transformation of the health system. Yet, for all this complexity, it is possible to measure progress, as a complement to the follow-up required for measuring progress towards universal coverage.

The first dimension to consider is the extent to which the organizational measures required to switch to primary care are being put into place.

- Is the predominant type of first-contact provider being shifted from specialists and hospitals to generalist primary-care teams in close proximity to where the people live?
- Are primary-care providers being made responsible for the health of all the members of a well-identified population: those who attend health services and those who do not?
- Are primary-care providers being empowered to coordinate the various inputs of specialized, hospital and social services, by strengthening their administrative authority and purchasing power?

The second dimension to consider is the extent to which the distinctive features of primary care are gaining prominence.

- Person-centredness: is there evidence of improvement, as shown by direct observation and user surveys?

- Comprehensiveness: is the portfolio of primary-care services expanding and becoming more comprehensive, reaching the full essential benefits package, from promotion through to palliation, for all age groups?
- Continuity: is information for individuals being recorded over the life-course, and transferred between levels of care in cases of referral and to a primary-care unit elsewhere when people relocate?
- Regular entry point: are measures taken to ensure that providers know their clients and vice versa?

This should provide the guidance to policy-makers as to the progress they are making with the transformation of health-care delivery. However, they do not immediately make it possible to attribute health and social outcomes to specific aspects of the reform efforts. In order to do so, the monitoring of the reform effort needs to be complemented with a much more vigorous research agenda. It is revealing that the Cochrane Review on strategies for integrating primary-health services in low- and middle-income countries could identify only one valid study that took the user's perspective into account[160]. There has been a welcome surge of research on primary care in high-income countries and, more recently, in the middle-income countries that have launched major PHC reforms. Nevertheless, it is remarkable that an industry that currently mobilizes 8.6% of the world's GDP invests so little in research on two of its most effective and cost-effective strategies: primary care and the public policies that underpin and complement it.

References

1. *People at the centre of health care: harmonizing mind and body, people and systems.* New Delhi, World Health Organization Regional Office for South-East Asia, Manila, World Health Organization Regional Office for the Western Pacific, 2007.
2. Osler W. *Aequanimitas*. Philadelphia PA, Blakiston, 1904.
3. Eby D. Primary care at the Alaska Native Medical Centre: a fully deployed "new model" of primary care. *International Journal of Circumpolar Health*, 2007, 66(Suppl. 1):4–13.
4. Eby D. Integrated primary care. *International Journal of Circumpolar Health*, 1998, 57(Suppl. 1):665–667.
5. Gottlieb K, Sylvester I, Eby D. Transforming your practice: what matters most. *Family Practice Management*, 2008, 15:32–38.
6. Kerssens JJ et al. Comparison of patient evaluations of health care quality in relation to WHO measures of achievement in 12 European countries. *Bulletin of the World Health Organization*, 2004 82:106–114.
7. Bossyns P, Miye M, Van Lerberghe W. Supply-level measures to increase uptake of family planning services in Niger: the effectiveness of improving responsiveness. *Tropical Medicine and International Health*, 2002, 7:383–390.
8. *The World Health Report 2000 – Health systems: improving performance*. Geneva, World Health Organization, 2000.
9. Mercer SW, Cawston PG, Bikker AP. Quality in general practice consultations: a qualitative study of the views of patients living in an area of high socio-economic deprivation in Scotland. *BMC Family Practice*, 2007, 8:22.
10. Scherger JE. What patients want. *Journal of Family Practice*, 2001, 50:137.
11. Sackett DL et al. Evidence based medicine: what it is and what it isn't. *British Medical Journal*, 1996, 312:71–72.
12. Guyatt G, Cook D, Haynes B. Evidence based medicine has come a long way: The second decade will be as exciting as the first. *BMJ*, 2004, 329:990–991.
13. Cochrane database of systematic reviews. The Cochrane Library, 2008 (http://www.cochrane.org, accessed 27 July 2008).
14. Iha A, ed. *Summary of the evidence on patient safety: implications for research*. Geneva, World Health Organization, The Research Priority Setting Working Group of the World Alliance for Patient Safety, 2008.
15. Smith GD, Mertens T. What's said and what's done: the reality of sexually transmitted disease consultations. *Public Health*, 2004, 118:96–103.
16. Berwick DM. The science of improvement. *JAMA*, 2008, 299:1182–1184.
17. Donaldson L, Philip P. Patient safety: a global priority. *Bulletin of the World Health Organization*, 2004, 82:892–893

18. Kohn LT, Corrigan JM, Donaldson MS, eds. *To err is human: building a safer health system*. Washington, DC, National Academy Press, Committee on Quality of Health Care in America, Institute of Medicine, 1999.
19. Reason J. Human error: models and management. *BMJ*, 2000, 320:768–770.
20. Kripalani S et al. Deficits in communication and information transfer between hospital-based and primary care physicians: implications for patient safety and continuity of care. *JAMA*, 2007, 297:831–841.
21. Miller MA, Pisani E. The cost of unsafe injections. *Bulletin of the World Health Organization*, 1999, 77:808–811.
22. *The purpose of a world alliance*. Geneva, World Health Organization, World Alliance for Patient Safety, 2008 (http://www.who.int/patientsafety/worldalliance/alliance/en/, accessed 28 July 2008).
23. Shortell SM, Singer SJ. Improving patient safety by taking systems seriously. *JAMA* 2008, 299:445–447.
24. Das J, Hammer JS, Kenneth LL. *The quality of medical advice in low-income countries*. Washington DC, The World Bank, 2008 (World Bank Policy Research Working Paper No. 4501; http://ssrn.com/abstract=1089272, accessed 28 Jul 2008).
25. Schoen C et al. Taking the pulse of health care systems: experiences of patients with health problems in six countries. *Health Affairs*, 2005 (web exclusive W 5-5 0 9 DOI 10.1377/hlthaff.W5.509).
26. Mekbib TA, Teferi B. Caesarean section and foetal outcome at Yekatit 12 hospital, Addis Abba, Ethiopia, 1987-1992. *Ethiopian Medical Journal*, 1994, 32:173–179.
27. Siddiqi S et al. The effectiveness of patient referral in Pakistan. *Health Policy and Planning*, 2001, 16:193–198.
28. Sanders D et al. Zimbabwe's hospital referral system: does it work? *Health Policy and Planning*, 1998, 13:359–370.
29. Data reported at World Aids Day Meeting, Antwerp, Belgium, 2000.
30. *The World Health Report 2005 – Make every mother and child count*. Geneva, World Health Organization, 2005.
31. Starfield B, Shi L, Macinko J. Contributions of primary care to health systems and health. *The Milbank Quarterly*, 2005, 83:457–502.
32. Heise L, Garcia-Moreno C. Intimate partner violence. In: Krug EG et al, eds. *World report on violence and health*. Geneva, World Health Organization, 2002.
33. Ellsberg M et al. Intimate partner violence and women's physical and mental health in the WHO multi-country study on women's health and domestic violence: an observational study. *Lancet*, 2008, 371:1165–1172.

34. Campbell JC. Health consequences of intimate partner violence. *Lancet*, 2002, 359:1331–1336.

35. Edleson JL. Children's witnessing of domestic violence. *Journal of Interpersonal Violence*, 1996, 14: 839–870.

36. Dube SR et al. Exposure to abuse, neglect, and household dysfunction among adults who witnessed intimate partner violence as children: implications for health and social services. *Violence and Victims*, 2002, 17: 3–17.

37. Åsling-Monemi K et al. Violence against women increases the risk of infant and child mortality: a case-referent study in Nicaragua. *Bulletin of the World Health Organization*, 2003, 81:10–18.

38. Bonomi A et al. Intimate partner violence and women's physical, mental and social functioning. *American Journal of Preventive Medicine*, 2006, 30:458-466.

39. National Centre for Injury Prevention and Control. *Costs of intimate partner violence against women in the United States*. Atlanta GA, Centres for Disease Control and Prevention, 2003.

40. Ramsay J et al. Should health professionals screen women for domestic violence? Systematic review. *BMJ*, 2002, 325:314–318.

41. Nelson HD et al. Screening women and elderly adults for family and intimate partner violence: a review of the evidence for the U.S. Preventive Services Task force. *Annals of Internal Medicine*, 2004, 140:387–403.

42. Garcia-Moreno C. Dilemmas and opportunities for an appropriate health-service response to violence against women. *Lancet*, 2002, 359:1509–1514.

43. Wathan NC, MacMillan HL. Interventions for violence against women. Scientific review. *JAMA*, 2003, 289:589–600.

44. Sullivan CM, Bybee DI. Reducing violence using community-based advocacy for women with abusive partners. *Journal of Consulting and Clinical Psychology*, 1999, 67:43–53.

45. Tiwari A et al. A randomized controlled trial of empowerment training for Chinese abused pregnant women in Hong Kong. *British Journal of Obstetrics and Gynaecology*, 2005, 112:1249–1256.

46. Taket A et al. Routinely asking women about domestic violence in health settings. *BMJ*, 2003, 327:673–676.

47. MacDonald R. Time to talk about rape. *BMJ*, 2000, 321:1034–1035.

48. Basile KC, Hertz FM, Back SE. *Intimate partner and sexual violence victimization instruments for use in healthcare settings*. 2008. Atlanta GA, Centers for Disease Control and Prevention, 2008.

49. *Guidelines for the medico-legal care of victims of sexual violence*. Geneva, World Health Organization, 2003.

50. Mead N, Bower P. Patient-centredness: a conceptual framework and review of the empirical literature. *Social Science and Medicine*, 51:1087–1110.

51. Stewart M. Towards a global definition of patient centred care. *BMJ*, 2001, 322:444–445.

52. Fiscella K et al. Patient trust: is it related to patient-centred behavior of primary care physicians? *Medical Care*, 2004, 42:1049–1055.

53. Marincowitz GJO, Fehrsen GS. *Caring, learning, improving quality and doing research: Different faces of the same process*. Paper presented at: 11th South African Family Practice Congress, Sun City, South Africa, August 1998.

54. Ferrer RL, Hambidge SJ, Maly RC. The essential role of generalists in health care systems. *Annals of Internal Medicine*, 2005, 142:691–699.

55. Gulbrandsen P, Hjortdahl P, Fugelli P. General practitioners' knowledge of their patients' psychosocial problems: multipractice questionnaire survey. *British Medical Journal*, 1997, 314:1014–1018.

56. Jaturapatporn D, Dellow A. Does family medicine training in Thailand affect patient satisfaction with primary care doctors? *BMC Family Practice*, 2007, 8:14.

57. Kovess-Masféty V et al. What makes people decide who to turn to when faced with a mental health problem? Results from a French survey. *BMC Public Health*, 2007, 7:188.

58. Bergeson D. A systems approach to patient-centred care. *JAMA*, 2006, 296:23.

59. Kravitz RL et al. Recall of recommendations and adherence to advice among patients with chronic medical conditions. *Archives of Internal Medicine*, 1993, 153:1869–1878.

60. Werner D et al. *Questioning the solution: the politics of primary health care and child survival, with an in-depth critique of oral rehydration therapy*. Palo Alto CA, Health Wrights, 1997.

61. Norris et al. Increasing diabetes self-management education in community settings. A systematic review. *American Journal of Preventive Medicine*, 2002, 22:39–66.

62. Bossyns P, Van Lerberghe W. The weakest link: competence and prestige as constraints to referral by isolated nurses in rural Niger. *Human Resources for Health*, 2004, 2:1.

63. Willems S et al. Socio-economic status of the patient and doctor-patient communication: does it make a difference. *Patient Education and Counseling*, 2005, 56:139–146.

64. Pongsupap Y. *Introducing a human dimension to Thai health care: the case for family practice*. Brussels, Vrije Universiteit Brussel Press. 2007.

65. *Renewing primary health care in the Americas. A Position paper of the Pan American Health Organization*. Washington DC, Pan American Health Organization, 2007.

66. Penny Simkin, PT. Birth plans: after 25 years, women still want to be heard. *Birth*, 34:49–51.

67. Portela A, Santarelli C. Empowerment of women, men, families and communities: true partners for improving maternal and newborn health. *British Medical Bulletin*, 2003, 67:59–72.

68. Wallerstein N. *What is the evidence on effectiveness of empowerment to improve health?* Copenhagen, World Health Organization Regional Office for Europe 2006 (Health Evidence Network report; (http://www.euro.who.int/Document/E88086.pdf, accessed 21-11-07).

69. Diabète-France.com – portail du diabète et des diabetiques en France, 2008 (http://www.diabete-france.com, accessed 30 July 2008).

70. Barlow J, Cohen E, Stewart-Brown SSB. Parent training for improving maternal psychosocial health. *Cochrane Database of Systematic Reviews*,2003, (4):CD002020.

71. Ahluwalia I. An evaluation of a community-based approach to safe motherhood in northwestern Tanzania. *International Journal of Gynecology and Obstetrics*, 2003, 82:231.

72. De la Luz Martínez-Maldonado M, Correa-Muñoz E, Mendoza-Núñez VM. Program of active aging in a rural Mexican community: a qualitative approach. *BMC Public Health*, 2007, 7:276 (DOI:10.1186/1471-2458-7-276).

73. Frenz P. *Innovative practices for intersectoral action on health: a case study of four programs for social equity*. Chilean case study prepared for the CSDH. Santiago, Ministry of Health, Division of Health Planning, Social Determinants of Health Initiative, 2007.

74. Paetthayasapaa. Kam Prakard Sitti Pu Paui, 2003? (http://www.tmc.or.th/, accessed 30 July 2008).

75. Prince M, Livingston G, Katona C. Mental health care for the elderly in low-income countries: a health systems approach. *World Psychiatry*, 2007, 6:5–13.

76. Nanda P. Women's participation in rural credit programmes in Bangladesh and their demand for formal health care: is there a positive impact? *Health Economics*, 1999, 8:415–428.

77. Nakkash R et al. The development of a feasible community-specific cardiovascular disease prevention program: triangulation of methods and sources. *Health Education and Behaviour*, 2003, 30:723–739.

78. Stange KC. The paradox of the parts and the whole in understanding and improving general practice. *International Journal for Quality in Health Care*, 2002, 14:267–268.

79. Gill JM. The structure of primary care: framing a big picture. *Family Medicine*, 2004, 36:65–68.

80. *Pan-Canadian Primary Health Care Indicator Development Project. Pan-Canadian primary health care indicators, Report 1, Volume 1.* Ottawa, Canadian Institute for Health Information 2008 (http:\www.cihi.ca).

81. Bindman AB et al. Primary care and receipt of preventive services. *Journal of General Internal Medicine*, 1996, 11:269–276.

82. Forrest CB, Starfield B. The effect of first-contact care with primary care clinicians on ambulatory health care expenditures. *Journal of Family Practice*, 1996, 43:40–48.

83. Chande VT, Kinane JM. Role of the primary care provider in expediting children with acute appendicitis. *Achives of Pediatrics and Adolescent Medicine*, 1996, 150:703–706.

84. Starfield B. *Primary care: balancing health needs, services, and technology*. New York, Oxford University Press 1998.

85. Bindman AB et al. Primary care and receipt of preventive services. *Journal of General Internal Medicine*, 1996, 11:269–276.

86. Shea S et al. Predisposing factors for severe, uncontrolled hypertension in an inner-city minority population. *New England Journal of Medicine*, 1992, 327:776–781.

87. Galobardes B, Lynch JW, Davey Smith G. Is the association between childhood socioeconomic circumstances and cause-specific mortality established? Update of a systematic review. *Journal of Epidemiology and Community Health*, 2008, 62:387–390.

88. *Guide to clinical preventive services, 2007*. Rockville MD, Agency for Healthcare Research and Quality, 2007 (AHRQ Publication No. 07-05100; http://www.ahrq.gov/clinic/pocketgd.htm).

89. Porignon D et al. *Comprehensive is effective: vaccination coverage and health system performance in Sub-Saharan Africa*, 2008 (forthcoming).

90. Shi L et al. The relationship between primary care, income inequality, and mortality in the United States, 1980–1995. *Journal of the American Board of Family Practice*, 2003, 16:412–422.

91. Franks P, Fiscella K. Primary care physicians and specialists as personal physicians. Health care expenditures and mortality experience. *Journal of Family Practice*, 1998, 47:105–109.

92. Villalbi JR et al. An evaluation of the impact of primary care reform on health. *Atenci'on Primaria*, 1999, 24:468–474.

93. *Regional core health data initiative.* Washington DC, Pan American Health Organization, 2006 (http://www.paho.org/English/SHA/corodata/tabulator/newTabulator.htm).

94. Weinick RM, Krauss NA. Racial/ethnic differences in children's access to care. *American Journal of Public Health*, 2000, 90:1771–1774.

95. Forrest CB, Starfield B. Entry into primary care and continuity: the effects of access. *American Journal of Public Health*, 1998, 88:1330–1336.

96. Weinberger M, Oddone EZ, Henderson WG. Does increased access to primary care reduce hospital readmissions? For The Veterans Affairs Cooperative Study Group on Primary Care and Hospital Readmission. *New England Journal of Medicine*, 1996, 334:1441–1447.

97. Woodward CA et al. What is important to continuity in home care? Perspectives of key stakeholders. *Social Science and Medicine*, 2004, 58:177–192.

98. Gill JM, Mainous AGI, Nsereko M. The effect of continuity of care on emergency department use. *Archives of Family Medicine*, 2000, 9:333–338.

99. Rothwell P. Subgroup analysis in randomised controlled trials: importance, indications, and interpretation, *Lancet*, 2005, 365:176–186.

100. Kravitz RL, Duan N, Braslow J. Evidence-based medicine, heterogeneity of treatment effects, and the trouble with averages. *The Milbank Quarterly*, 2004, 82:661–687.

101. Stiell A. et al. Prevalence of information gaps in the emergency department and the effect on patient outcomes. *Canadian Medical Association Journal*, 2003, 169:1023–1028.

102. Smith PC et al. Missing clinical information during primary care visits. *JAMA*, 2005, 293:565–571.

103. Elder NC, Vonder Meulen MB, Cassedy A. The identification of medical errors by family physicians during outpatient visits. *Annals of Family Medicine*, 2004, 2:125–129.

104. Elwyn G. Safety from numbers: identifying drug related morbidity using electronic records in primary care. *Quality and Safety in Health Care*, 2004, 13:170–171.

105. Open Medical Records System (OpenMRS) [online database]. Cape Town, South African Medical Research Council, 2008 (http://openmrs.org/wiki/OpenMRS, accessed 29 July 2008).

106. Hüsler J, Peters T. *Evaluation of the On Cue Compliance Service pilot: testing the use of SMS reminders in the treatment of tuberculosis in Cape Town, South Africa. Prepared for the City of Cape Town Health Directorate and the International Development Research Council (IDRC).* Cape Town, Bridges Organization, 2005.

107. Smith-Rohrberg Maru D et al. Poor follow-up rates at a self-pay northern Indian tertiary AIDS clinic. *International Journal for Equity in Health*, 2007, 6:14.

108. Busse R, Schlette S, eds. *Focus on prevention, health and aging, and health professions.* Gütersloh, Verlag Bertelsmann Stiftung, 2007 (Health policy developments 7/8).

109. James Pfeiffer International. NGOs and primary health care in Mozambique: the need for a new model of collaboration. *Social Science and Medicine*, 2003, 56:725–738.

110. Jaffré Y, Olivier de Sardan J-P. *Une médecine inhospitalière. Les difficiles relations entre soignants et soignés dans cinq capitales d'Afrique de l'Ouest.* Paris, Karthala, 2003.

111. Naithani S, Gulliford M, Morgan M. Patients' perceptions and experiences of "continuity of care" in diabetes. *Health Expectations*, 2006, 9:118–129.

112. Schoenbaum SC. The medical home: a practical way to improve care and cut costs. *Medscape Journal of Medicine* , 2007, 9:28.

113. Beach MC. Are physicians' attitudes of respect accurately perceived by patients and associated with more positive communication behaviors? *Patient Education and Counselling*, 2006, 62:347–354 (Epub 2006 Jul 21).

114. Farmer JE et al. Comprehensive primary care for children with special health care needs in rural areas. *Pediatrics*, 2005, 116:649–656.

115. Pongsupap Y, Van Lerberghe W. Patient experience with self-styled family practices and conventional primary care in Thailand. *Asia Pacific Family Medicine Journal*, 2006, Vol 5.

116. Weiss LJ, Blustein J. Faithful patients: the effect of long term physician–patient relationships on the costs and use of health care by older Americans. *American Journal of Public Health*, 1996, 86:1742–1747.

117. Rosenblatt RL et al. The generalist role of specialty physicians: is there a hidden system of primary care? *JAMA*,1998, 279:1364–1370.

118. Kempe A et al. Quality of care and use of the medical home in a state-funded capitated primary care plan for low-income children. *Pediatrics*, 2000, 105:1020–1028.

119. Raddish MS et al. Continuity of care: is it cost effective? *American Journal of Managed Care*, 1999, 5:727–734.

120. De Maeseneer JM et al. Provider continuity in family medicine: does it make a difference for total health care costs? *Annals of Family Medicine*, 2003, 1:131–133.

121. Saver B. Financing and organization findings brief. *Academy for Research and Health Care Policy*, 2002, 5:1–2.

122. Tudiver F, Herbert C, Goel V. Why don't family physicians follow clinical practice guidelines for cancer screening? *Canadian Medical Association Journal*, 1998, 159:797–798.

123. Oxman AD et al. No magic bullets: a systematic review of 102 trials of interventions to improve professional practice. *Canadian Medical Association Journal*, 1995, 153:1423–1431.

124. Freeman G, Hjortdahl P. What future for continuity of care in general practice? *British Medical Journal*, 1997, 314: 1870–1873.

125. Miller MR et al. Parental preferences for primary and specialty care collaboration in the management of teenagers with congenital heart disease. *Pediatrics*, 2000, 106:264–269.

126. Mainous AG III, Gill JM. The importance of continuity of care in the likelihood of future hospitalization: is site of care equivalent to a primary clinician? *American Journal of Public Health*, 1998, 88:1539–1541.

127. Parchman ML, Culler SD. Primary care physicians and avoidable hospitalizations. *Journal of Family Practice*, 1994, 39:123–128.

128. Hurley RE, Freund DA, Taylor DE. Emergency room use and primary care case management: evidence from four medicaid demonstration programs. *American Journal of Public Health*, 1989, 79: 834–836.

129. Martin DP et al. Effect of a gatekeeper plan on health services use and charges: a randomized trial. *American Journal of Public Health*, 1989, 79:1628–1632.

130. Gadomski A, Jenkins P, Nichols M. Impact of a Medicaid Primary Care Provider and Preventive Care on pediatric hospitalization. *Pediatrics*, 1998, 101:E1 (http://pediatrics.aappublications.org/cgi/reprint/101/3/e1, accessed 29 July 2008).

131. Hjortdahl P, Borchgrevink CF. Continuity of care: influence of general practitioners' knowledge about their patients on use of resources in consultations. *British Medical Journal*, 1991, 303:1181–1184.

132. Roos NP, Carriere KC, Friesen D. Factors influencing the frequency of visits by hypertensive patients to primary care physicians in Winnipeg. *Canadian Medical Association Journal*, 1998, 159:777–783.

133. Ryan S et al. The effects of regular source of care and health need on medical care use among rural adolescents. *Archives of Pediatric and Adolescent Medicine*, 2001, 155:184–190.

134. Schoen C et al. Towards higher-performance health systems: adults' health care experiences in seven countries, 2007. *Health Affairs*, 2007, 26:w717–w734.

135. Saltman R, Rico A, Boerma W, eds. *Primary care in the driver's seat? Organizational reform in European primary care.* Maidenhead, England, Open University Press, 2006 (European Observatory on Health Systems and Policies Series).

136. Nutting PA. Population-based family practice: the next challenge of primary care. *Journal of Family Practice*, 1987, 24:83–88.

137. *Strategies for population health: investing in the health of Canadians.* Ottawa, Health Canada, Advisory Committee on Population Health, 1994.

138. Lasker R. *Medicine and public health: the power of collaboration.* New York, New York Academy of Medicine, 1997.

139. Longlett SK, Kruse JE, Wesley RM. Community-oriented primary care: historical perspective. *Journal of the American Board of Family Practice*, 2001,14:54–563.

140. *Improving health for New Zealanders by investing in primary health care.* Wellington, National Health Committee, 2000.

141. Provenzale D et al. Gastroenterologist specialist care and care provided by generalists – an evaluation of effectiveness and efficiency. *American Journal of Gastroenterology*, 2003, 98:21-8.

142. Smetana GW et al. A comparison of outcomes resulting from generalist vs specialist care for a single discrete medical condition: a systematic review and methodologic critique. *Archives of Internal Medicine*, 2007, 167:10–20.

143. Beck CA et al. Discharge prescriptions following admission for acute myocardial infarction at tertiary care and community hospitals in Quebec. *Canadian Journal of Cardiology*, 2001, 17:33–40.

144. Fendrick AM, Hirth RA, Chernew ME. Differences between generalist and specialist physicians regarding Helicobacter pylori and peptic ulcer disease. *American Journal of Gastroenterology*, 1996, 91:1544–1548.

145. Zoorob RJ et al. Practice patterns for peptic ulcer disease: are family physicians testing for H. pylori? *Helicobacter*, 1999, 4:243–248.

146. Rose JH et al. Generalists and oncologists show similar care practices and outcomes for hospitalized late-stage cancer patients. For SUPPORT Investigators (Study to Understand Prognoses and Preferences for Outcomes and Risks for Treatment). *Medical Care*, 2000, 38:1103–1118.

147. Krikke EH, Bell NR. Relation of family physician or specialist care to obstetric interventions and outcomes in patients at low risk: a western Canadian cohort study. *Canadian Medical Association Journal*, 1989, 140:637–643.

148. MacDonald SE, Voaklander K, Birtwhistle RV. A comparison of family physicians' and obstetricians' intrapartum management of low-risk pregnancies. *Journal of Family Practice*, 1993, 37:457-462.

149. Abyad A, Homsi R. A comparison of pregnancy care delivered by family physicians versus obstetricians in Lebanon. *Family Medicine*, 1993 25:465–470.

150. Grunfeld E et al. Comparison of breast cancer patient satisfaction with follow-up in primary care versus specialist care: results from a randomized controlled trial. *British Journal of General Practice*, 1999, 49:705–710.

151. Grunfeld E et al. Randomized trial of long-term follow-up for early-stage breast cancer: a comparison of family physician versus specialist care. *Journal of Clinical Oncology*, 2006, 24:848–855.

152. Scott IA et al. An Australian comparison of specialist care of acute myocardial infarction. *International Journal for Quality in Health Care*, 2003, 15:155–161..

153. Regueiro CR et al. A comparison of generalist and pulmonologist care for patients hospitalized with severe chronic obstructive pulmonary disease: resource intensity, hospital costs, and survival. For SUPPORT Investigators (Study to Understand Prognoses and Preferences for Outcomes and Risks of Treatment). *American Journal of Medicine*, 1998, 105:366–372.

154. McAlister FA et al. The effect of specialist care within the first year on subsequent outcomes in 24,232 adults with new-onset diabetes mellitus: population-based cohort study. *Quality and Safety in Health Care*, 2007, 16:6–11.

155. Greenfield S et al. Outcomes of patients with hypertension and non-insulin dependent diabetes mellitus treated by different systems and specialties. Results from the medical outcomes study. *Journal of the American Medical Association*, 1995, 274:1436–1444.

156. Pongsupap Y, Boonyapaisarnchoaroen T, Van Lerberghe W. The perception of patients using primary care units in comparison with conventional public hospital outpatient departments and "prime mover family practices": an exit survey. *Journal of Health Science*, 2005, 14:3.

157. Baicker K, Chandra A. Medicare spending, the physician workforce, and beneficiaries' quality of care. *Health Affairs*, 2004 (Suppl. web exclusive: W4-184–197).

158. Shi, L. Primary care, specialty care, and life chances. *International Journal of Health Services*, 1994, 24:431–458.

159. Baicker K et al. Who you are and where you live: how race and geography affect the treatment of Medicare beneficiaries. *Health Affairs*, 2004 (web exclusive: VAR33–V44).

160. Briggs CJ, Garner P. Strategies for integrating primary health services in middle and low-income countries at the point of delivery. *Cochrane Database of Systematic Reviews*, 2006, (3):CD003318.

161. *Estudo regional sobre assistencia hospitalar e ambulatorial especializada na America Latina e Caribe*. Washington DC, Pan American Health Organization, Unidad de Organización de Servicios de Salud, Area de Tecnología y Prestación de Servicios de Salud, 2004.

162. Pongsupap Y, Van Lerberghe W. Choosing between public and private or between hospital and primary care? Responsiveness, patient-centredness and prescribing patterns in outpatient consultations in Bangkok. *Tropical Medicine and International Health*, 2006, 11:81–89.

163. *Guide to clinical preventive services, 2007*. Rockville MD, Agency for Healthcare Research and Quality, 2007 (AHRQ Publication No. 07-05100; http://www.ahrq.gov/clinic/pocketgd.htm).

164. Margolis PA et al. From concept to application: the impact of a community-wide intervention to improve the delivery of preventive services to children. *Pediatrics*, 2001, 108:E42.

165. Donovan EF et al. Intensive home visiting is associated with decreased risk of infant death. *Pediatrics*, 2007, 119:1145–1151.

166. Manandhar D et al. Effect of a participatory intervention with women's groups on birth outcomes in Nepal: cluster-randomised controlled trial. *Lancet*, 364:970–979.

167. Rockenschaub G, Pukkila J, Profili MC, eds. *Towards health security. A discussion paper on recent health crises in the WHO European Region*. Copenhagen, World Health Organization Regional Office for Europe, 2007

168. *Primary care. America's health in a new era*. Washington DC, National Academy Press Institute of Medicine, 1996.

169. Tableau d'honneur des 50 meilleurs hôpitaux de France. Palmarès des Hôpitaux. *Le Point*, 2008 (http://hopitaux.lepoint.fr/tableau-honneur.php, accessed 29 July 2008).

170. Davidson BN, Sofaer S, Gertler P. Consumer information and biased selection in the demand for coverage supplementing Medicare. *Social Science and Medicine*, 1992, 34:1023–1034.

171. Davison KP, Pennebaker JW, Dickerson SS. Who talks? The social psychology of illness support groups. *American Psychology*, 2000, 55:205–217.

172. Segal SP, Redman D, Silverman C. Measuring clients' satisfaction with self-help agencies. *Psychiatric Services*, 51:1148–1152.

173. Adapted from Wollast E, Mercenier P. Pour une régionalisation des soins. In: Groupe d'Etude pour une Réforme de la Médecine. *Pour une politique de la santé*. Bruxelles, Editions Vie Ouvrière/La Revue Nouvelle, 1971.

174. Criel B, De Brouwere V, Dugas S. *Integration of vertical programmes in multi-function health services*. Antwerp, ITGPress, 1997 (Studies in Health Services Organization and Policy 3).

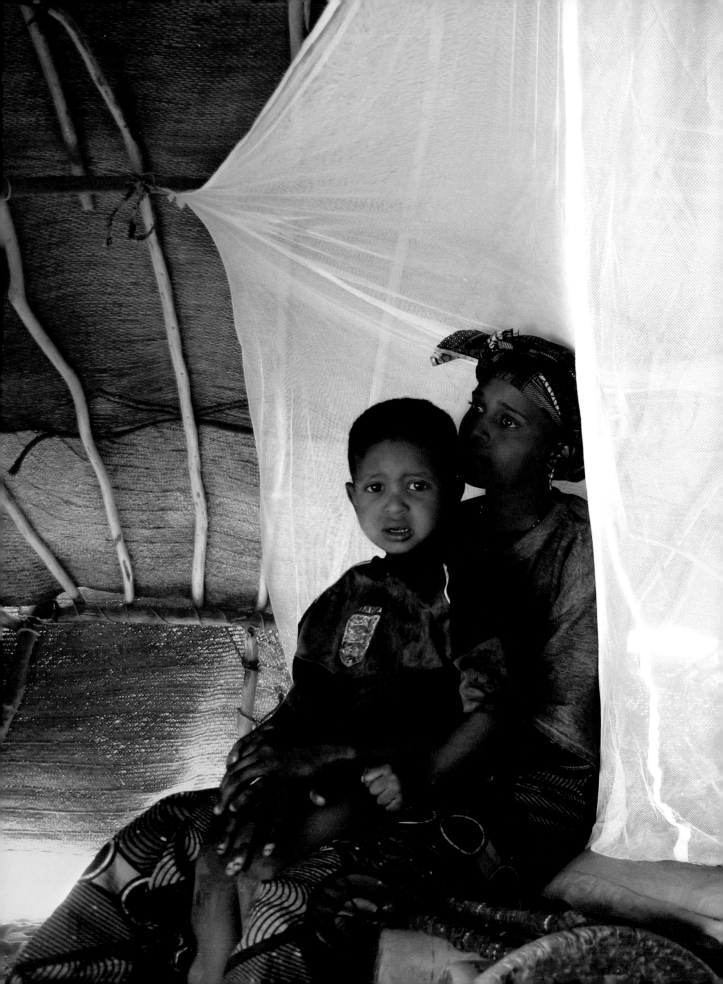

Public policies
for the public's health

◆◆ *Public policies in the health sector, together with those in other sectors, have a huge potential to secure the health of communities. They represent an important complement to universal coverage and service delivery reforms. Unfortunately, in most societies, this potential is largely untapped and failures to effectively engage other sectors are widespread. Looking ahead at the diverse range of challenges associated with the growing importance of ageing, urbanization and the social determinants of health, there is, without question, a need for a greater capacity to seize this potential. That is why a drive for better public policies – the theme of this chapter – forms a third pillar supporting the move towards PHC, along with universal coverage and primary care.*

Chapter 4

The chapter reviews the policies that must be in place. These are:

- systems policies – the arrangements that are needed across health systems' building blocks to support universal coverage and effective service delivery;
- public-health policies – the specific actions needed to address priority health problems through cross-cutting prevention and health promotion; and
- policies in other sectors – contributions to health that can be made through intersectoral collaboration.

The chapter explains how these different public policies can be strengthened and aligned with the goals pursued by PHC.

The importance of effective public policies for health

People want to live in communities and environments which secure and promote their health[1]. Primary care, with universal access and social protection represent key responses to these expectations. People also expect their governments to put into place an array of public policies that span local through to supra-national level arrangements, without which primary care and universal coverage lose much of their impact and meaning. These include the policies required to make health systems function properly; to organize public-health actions of major benefit to all; and, beyond the health sector, the policies that can contribute to health and a sense of security, while ensuring that issues, such as urbanization, climate change, gender discrimination or social stratification are properly addressed.

A first group of critical public policies are the health systems policies (related to essential drugs, technology, quality control, human resources, accreditation, etc.) on which primary care and universal coverage reforms depend. Without functional supply and logistics systems, for example, a primary-care network cannot function properly: in Kenya, for example, children are now much better protected against malaria as a result of local services providing them with insecticide-treated bednets[2]. This has only been possible because the work of primary care was supported by a national initiative with strong political commitment, social marketing and national support for supply and logistics.

Effective public-health policies that address priority health problems are a second group without which primary care and universal coverage reforms would be hindered. These encompass the technical policies and programmes that provide guidance to primary-care teams on how to deal with priority health problems. They also encompass the classical public-health interventions, from public hygiene and disease prevention to health promotion. Some interventions, such as the fortification of salt with iodine, are only feasible at the regional, national or, increasingly at supra-national level. This may be because it is only at those levels that there is the necessary authority to decide upon such policies, or because it is more efficient to develop and implement such policies on a scale that is beyond the local dimensions of primary-care action. Finally, public policies encompass the rapid response capacity, in command-and-control mode, to deal with acute threats to the public's health, particularly epidemics and catastrophes. The latter is of the utmost political importance, because failures profoundly affect the public's trust in its health authorities. The lack of preparedness and uncoordinated responses of both the Canadian and the Chinese health systems to the outbreak of SARS in 2003, led to public outcries and eventually to the establishment of a national public health agency in Canada. In China, a similar lack of preparedness and transparency led to a crisis in confidence – a lesson learned in time for subsequent events[3,4].

The third set of policies that is of critical concern is known as "health in all policies", which is based on the recognition that population health can be improved through policies that are mainly controlled by sectors other than health[5]. The health content of school curricula, industry's policy towards gender equality, or the safety of food and consumer goods are all issues that can profoundly influence or even determine the health of entire communities, and that can cut across national boundaries. It is not possible to address such issues without intensive intersectoral collaboration that gives due weight to health in all policies.

Better public policies can make a difference in very different ways. They can mobilize the whole of society around health issues, as in Cuba (Box 4.1). They can provide a legal and social environment that is more or less favourable to health outcomes. The degree of legal access to abortion, for example, co-determines the frequency and related mortality of unsafe abortion[6]. In South Africa, a change in legislation increased women's access to a broad range of options for the prevention and treatment of unwanted pregnancy, resulting in a 91% drop in abortion-related deaths[7]. Public policies can anticipate future problems. In Bangladesh, for example, the death toll due to high intensity cyclones and flooding was 240 000 people in 1970. With emergency preparedness and multisectoral risk reduction programmes, the death toll of comparable or more severe storms was reduced to 138 000 people in 1991 and 4500 people in 2007[8,9,10].

In the 23 developing countries that comprise 80% of the global chronic disease burden, 8.5 million lives could be saved in a decade by a 15% dietary salt reduction through manufacturers voluntarily reducing salt content in processed foods and a sustained mass-media campaign encouraging dietary change. Implementation of four measures from the Framework Convention on Tobacco Control (increased tobacco taxes;

smoke-free workplaces; convention-compliant packaging, labelling and awareness campaigns about health risks; and a comprehensive advertising, promotion, and sponsorship ban) could save a further 5.5 million lives in a decade[11]. As is often the case when considering social, economic and political determinants of ill-health, improvements are dependent on a fruitful collaboration between the health sector and a variety of other sectors.

Box 4.1 Rallying society's resources for health in Cuba[14,15,16]

In Cuba, average life expectancy at birth is the second highest in the Americas: in 2006, it was 78 years, and only 7.1 per 1000 children died before the age of five. Educational indicators for young children are among the best in Latin America. Cuba has achieved these results despite significant economic difficulties – even today, GDP per capita is only I$ 4500. Cuba's success in ensuring child welfare reflects its commitment to national public-health action and intersectoral action.

The development of human resources for health has been a national priority. Cuba has a higher proportion of doctors in the population than any other country. Training for primary care gives specific attention to the social determinants of health. They work in multidisciplinary teams in comprehensive primary-care facilities, where they are accountable for the health of a geographically defined population providing both curative and preventive services. They work in close contact with their communities, social services and schools, reviewing the health of all children twice a year with the teachers. They also work with organizations such as the Federation of Cuban Women (FMC) and political structures. These contacts provide them with the means to act on the social determinants of health within their communities.

Cuban national policy has also prioritized investing in early child development. There are three non-compulsory pre-school education programmes, which together are taken up by almost 100% of children under six years of age. In these programmes, screening for developmental disorders facilitates early intervention. Children who are identified with special needs, and their families, receive individual attention through multidisciplinary teams that contain both health and educational specialists. National policy in Cuba has not succumbed to a false choice between investing in the medical workforce and acting on the social determinants of health. Instead, it has promoted intersectoral cooperation to improve health through a strong preventive approach. In support of this policy, a large workforce has been trained to be competent in clinical care, working as an active part of the community it serves.

Figure 4.1 Deaths attributable to unsafe abortion per 100 000 live births, by legal grounds for abortion[a,12,13]

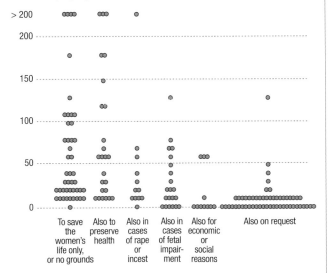

[a]Every dot represents one country.

System policies that are aligned with PHC goals

There is growing awareness that when parts of the health system malfunction, or are misaligned, the overall performance suffers. Referred to variously as "core functions"[17] or "building blocks"[18], the components of health systems include infrastructure, human resources, information, technologies and financing – all with consequences for the provision of services. These components are not aligned naturally or simply with the intended direction of PHC reforms that promote primary care and universal coverage: to obtain that alignment requires deliberate and comprehensive policy arrangements.

Experience in promoting essential medicines has shed light on both the opportunities and obstacles to effective systems policies for PHC. Since the *WHO List of Essential Medicines* was established in 1977, it has become a primary stimulus to the development of national medicines policies. Over 75% of the 193 WHO Member States now claim to have a national list of essential medicines, and over 100 countries have developed a national medicine policy. Surveys reveal that these policies have been effective in making lower cost and safer medicines available and more rationally used[19,20]. This particular policy has been successfully designed to support PHC, and it offers lessons on how to handle cross-cutting challenges of scale efficiencies and systems co-dependence. Without such arrangements, the health costs are enormous: nearly 30 000 children die every day from diseases that could easily have been treated if they had had access to essential medicines[21].

Medicines policies are indicative of how efficiencies in the scale of organization can be tapped. Safety, efficacy and quality of care have universal properties that make them amenable to globally agreed international standards. Adoption and adaptation of these global standards by national authorities is much more efficient than each country inventing its own standards. National decision-making and purchasing mechanisms can then guide rational, cost-effectiveness-based selection of medicines and reduce costs through bulk purchase. For example, Figure 4.2 shows how centralized oversight of drug purchasing

and subsidization in New Zealand significantly improved access to essential medicines while lowering the average prescription price. On a larger scale, transnational mechanisms, such as UNICEF's international procurement of vaccines, PAHO's Revolving Fund and the Global Drug Facility for tuberculosis treatment, afford considerable savings as well as quality assurances that countries on their own would be unlikely to negotiate[22,23,24,25].

A second key lesson of experience with essential drugs policies is that a policy cannot exist as an island and expect to be effectively implemented. Its formulation must identify those other systems elements, be they financing, information, infrastructure or human resources, upon which its implementation is dependent. Procurement mechanisms for pharmaceuticals, for example, raise important considerations for systems financing policies: they are interdependent. Likewise, human resources issues related to the education of consumers as well as the training and working conditions of providers are likely to be key determinants of the rational use of drugs.

Systems policies for human resources have long been a neglected area and one of the main constraints to health systems development[27]. The realization that the health MDGs are contingent on bridging the massive health-worker shortfall in low-income countries has brought long overdue attention to a previously neglected area. Furthermore, the evidence of increasing dependence on migrant health workers to address shortages in OECD countries underlines the fact that one country's policies may have a significant impact on another's. The choices countries make – or fail to

Figure 4.2 Annual pharmaceutical spending and number of prescriptions dispensed in New Zealand since the Pharmaceutical Management Agency was convened in 1993[26]

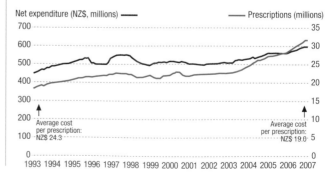

make – can have major long-term consequences. Human resources for health are the indispensable input to effective implementation of primary care and universal coverage reforms, and they are also the personification of the values that define PHC. Yet, in the absence of a deliberate choice to guide the health workforce policy by the PHC goals, market forces within the health-care system will drive health workers towards greater sub-specialization in tertiary care institutions, if not towards migration to large cities or other countries. PHC-based policy choices, on the other hand, focus on making staff available for the extension of coverage to underserved areas and disadvantaged population groups, as with Malaysia's scaling up of 11 priority cadres of workers, Ethiopia's training of 30 000 Health Extension Workers, Zambia's incentives to health workers to serve in rural areas, the 80 000 Lady Health Workers in Pakistan, or the task shifting for the care of HIV patients. These policies direct investments towards the establishment of the primary-care teams that are to be the hub of the PHC-based health system: the 80 000 health workers for Brazil's 30 000 Family Health Teams or the retraining of over 10 000 nurses and physicians in Turkey. Furthermore, these policies require both financial and non-financial incentives to compete effectively for scarce human resources, as in the United Kingdom, where measures have been taken to make a career in primary care financially competitive with specialization.

The core business of ministries of health and other public authorities is to put into place, across the various building blocks of the health system, the set of arrangements and mechanisms required to meet their health goals. When a country chooses to base its health systems on PHC – when it starts putting into place primary care and universal coverage reforms – its whole arsenal of system policies needs to be aligned behind these reforms: not just those pertaining to service delivery models or financing. It is possible to develop system policies that do not take account of the PHC agenda. It is also possible to choose to align them to PHC. If a country opts for PHC, effective implementation allows no half measures; no health systems building block will be left untouched.

Public-health policies

Aligning priority health programmes with PHC

Much action in the health sector is marshalled around specific high-burden diseases, such as HIV/AIDS, or stages of the life course such as children – so-called priority health conditions. The health programmes that are designed around these priorities are often comprehensive insofar as they set norms, ensure visibility and quality assurance, and entail a full range of entry points to address them locally or at the level of countries or regions. Responses to these priority health conditions can be developed in ways that either strengthen or undercut PHC[28].

In 1999 for example, the Primary Care Department of the Brazilian Paediatrics Society (SBP) prepared a plan to train its members in the Integrated Management of Childhood Illness (IMCI) and to adapt this strategy to regional epidemiological characteristics[29]. Despite conducting an initial training course, the SBP then warned paediatricians that IMCI was not a substitute for traditional paediatric care and risked breaching the basic rights of children and adolescents. In a next step, it objected to the delegation of tasks to the nurses, who are part of the multidisciplinary family health teams, the backbone of Brazil's PHC policy. Eventually, the SBP attempted to reclaim child and adolescent care as the exclusive domain of paediatricians with the argument that this ensured the best quality of care.

Experience with priority health programmes shows that the way they are designed makes the difference: trying to construct an entire set of PHC reforms around the unique requirements of a single disease leads to considerable inefficiencies. Yet, the reverse is equally true. While AIDS has been referred to as a metaphor for all that ails health systems and the wider society[30], the global response to the HIV pandemic can, in many respects, also be viewed as a pathfinder for PHC. From the start, it has had a strong rights-based and social justice foundation[31]. Its links to often marginalized and disadvantaged high-risk constituencies, and concerns about stigma, have led to concerted efforts to secure their rights and entitlements to employment, social services and health care. Efforts to scale-up services to conform to the goals of universal access have helped to expose the critical constraints deriving from the workforce crisis. The challenge of providing life-long treatment in resource-constrained settings has inspired innovations, such as more effective deployment of scarce human resources via "task shifting", the use of "patient advocates"[32], and the unexpected implementation of electronic health records. Most importantly, the adoption of a continuum of care approaches for HIV/AIDS from prevention to treatment to palliation has helped to revive and reinforce core features of primary care, such as comprehensiveness, continuity and person-centredness[32].

Countrywide public-health initiatives

While it is essential that primary-care teams seek to improve the health of populations at local level, this may be of limited value if national- and global-level policy-makers fail to take initiatives for broader, public policy measures, which are important in changing nutrition patterns and influencing the social determinants of health. These can rarely be implemented only in the context of local policies. Classical areas in which beyond-local-scale public-health interventions may be beneficial include: altering individual behaviours and lifestyles; controlling and preventing disease; tackling hygiene and the broader determinants of health; and secondary prevention, including screening for disease[33]. This includes measures such as the fortification of bread with folate, taxation of alcohol and tobacco, and ensuring the safety of food, consumer goods and toxic substances. Such national- and transnational-scale public-health interventions have the potential to save millions of lives. The successful removal of the major risk factors of disease, which is technically possible, would reduce premature deaths by an estimated 47% and increase global healthy life expectancy by an estimated 9.3 years[34]. However, as is the case for the priority programmes discussed above, the corresponding public-health policies must be designed so as to reinforce the PHC reforms.

Not all such public-health interventions will improve, for example, equity. Health promotion efforts that target individual risk behaviours,

such as health education campaigns aimed at smoking, poor nutrition and sedentary lifestyles, have often inadvertently exacerbated inequities. Socioeconomic differences in the uptake of one-size-fits-all public-health interventions have, at times, not only resulted in increased health inequities, but also in victim-blaming to explain the phenomenon[35]. Well-designed public-health policies can, however, reduce inequities when they provide health benefits to entire populations or when they explicitly prioritize groups with poor health[36]. The evidence base for privileging public policies that reduce inequities is increasing, most notably through the work of the Commission on Social Determinants of Health (Box 4.2)[37].

Rapid response capacity

While PHC reforms emphasize the importance of participatory and deliberative engagement of diverse stakeholders, humanitarian disasters or disease outbreaks demand a rapid response capacity that is crucial in dealing effectively with the problem at hand and is an absolute imperative in maintaining the trust of the population in their health system. Invoking quarantines or travel bans, rapidly sequencing the genome of a new pathogen to inform vaccine or therapeutic design, and mobilizing health workers and institutions without delay can be vital. While the advent of an "emergency" often provides the necessary good will and flexibility of these diverse actors to respond, an effective response is more likely if there have been significant investments in preparedness[38].

Global efforts related to the threat of pandemic avian influenza (H5N1) provide a number of interesting insights into how policies that inform preparedness and response could be guided by the values of PHC related to equity, universal coverage and primary-care reforms. In dealing with seasonal and pandemic influenza, 116 national influenza laboratories, and five international collaborating centre laboratories share influenza viruses in a system that was started by WHO over 50 years ago. The system was implemented to identify new pandemic virus threats and inform the optimal annual preparation of a seasonal influenza vaccine that is used primarily by industrialized countries. With the primarily

---

Box 4.2 Recommendations of the Commission on Social Determinants of Health[37]

The Commission on Social Determinants of Health (CSDH) was a three-year effort begun in 2005 to provide evidence-based recommendations for action on social determinants to reduce health inequities. The Commission accumulated an unprecedented collection of material to guide this process, drawing from theme-based knowledge networks, civil society experiences, country partners and departments within WHO. The final report of the CSDH contains a detailed series of recommendations for action, organized around the following three overarching recommendations.

1. Improve daily living conditions

Key improvements required in the well-being of girls and women; the circumstances in which their children are born; early child development and education for girls and boys; living and working conditions; social protection policy; and conditions for a flourishing older life.

2. Tackle the inequitable distribution of power, money and resources

To address health inequities it is necessary to address inequities in the way society is organized. This requires a strong public sector that is committed, capable and adequately financed. This in turn requires strengthened governance including stronger civil society and an accountable private sector. Governance dedicated to pursuing equity is required at all levels.

3. Measure and understand the problem and assess the impact of action

It is essential to acknowledge the problem of health inequity and ensure that it is measured – both within countries and globally. National and global health equity surveillance systems for routine monitoring of health inequity and the social determinants of health are required that also evaluate the health equity impact of policy and action. Other requirements are the training of policy-makers and health practitioners, increased public understanding of social determinants of health, and a stronger social determinants focus in research.

---

developing country focus of human zoonotic infections and the spectre of a global pandemic associated with H5N1 strains of influenza, the interest in influenza now extends to developing countries, and the long-standing public-private approach to influenza vaccine production and virus sharing has come under intense scrutiny. The expectation of developing countries for equitable access to protection, including affordable access to anti-virals and vaccines in the event of a pandemic, is resulting in changes to national and global capacity strengthening: from surveillance and laboratories to capacity transfer for vaccine formulation and production, and capacity for stock-piling. Thus, the most equitable response is the most effective response, and the most effective rapid response capacity can only emerge from the engagement of multiple stakeholders in this global process of negotiation.

Towards health in all policies

The health of populations is not merely a product of health sector activities – be they primary-care action or countrywide public-health action. It is to a large extent determined by societal and economic factors, and hence by policies and actions that are not within the remit of the health sector. Changes in the workplace, for example, can have a range of consequences for health (Table 4.1).

Confronted with these phenomena, the health authorities may perceive the sector as powerless to do more than try to mitigate the consequences. It cannot, of itself, redefine labour relations or unemployment arrangements. Neither can it increase taxes on alcohol, impose technical norms on motor vehicles or regulate rural migration and the development of slums – although all these measures can yield health benefits. Good urban governance, for example, can lead to 75 years or more of life expectancy, against as few as 35 years with poor governance[39]. Thus, it is important for the health sector to engage with other sectors, not just in order to obtain collaboration on tackling pre-identified priority health problems, as is the case for well-designed public-health interventions, but to ensure that health is recognized as one of the socially valued outcomes of all policies.

Such intersectoral action was a fundamental principle of the Alma-Ata Declaration. However, ministries of health in many countries have struggled to coordinate with other sectors or wield influence beyond the health system for which they are formally responsible. A major obstacle to reaping the rewards of intersectoral action has been the tendency, within the health sector, to see such collaboration as "mostly symbolic in trying to get other sectors to help [health] services"[40]. Intersectoral action has often not concentrated

Table 4.1 Adverse health effects of changing work circumstances[5]

Adverse health effects of unemployment	Adverse health effects of restructuring	Adverse health effects of non-standard work arrangements
Elevated blood pressure	Reduced job satisfaction, reduced organizational commitment and greater stress	Higher rates of occupational injury and disease than workers with full-time stable employment
Increased depression and anxiety		High level of stress, low job satisfaction and other negative health and well-being factors
Increased visits to general practitioners	Feelings of unfairness in downsizing process	More common in distributive and personal service sub-sectors where people in general have lower educational attainment and low skill levels
Increased symptoms of coronary disease	Survivors face new technologies, work processes, new physical and psychological exposures (reduced autonomy, increased work intensity, changes in the characteristics of social relationships, shifts in the employment contracts and changes in personal behaviour)	Low entitlement to workers' compensation and low level of claims by those who are covered
Worse mental health and greater stress		Increased occupational health hazards due to work intensification motivated by economic pressures
Increased psychological morbidity and increased medical visits		Inadequate training and poor communication caused by institutional disorganization and inadequate regulatory control
Decreased self-reported health status and an increase in the number of health problems	Changes in the psychological contract and lost sense of trust	Inability of workers to organize their own protection
	Prolonged stress with physiological and psychological signs	Cumulative trauma claims are difficult to show due to mobility of workers
Increase in family problems, particularly financial hardships		Reduced ability to improve life conditions due to inability to obtain credit, find housing, make pension arrangements, and possibility for training
		Fewer concerns for environmental issues and health and safety at work

on improving the policies of other sectors, but on instrumentalizing their resources: mobilizing teachers to contribute to the distribution of bednets, police officers to trace tuberculosis treatment defaulters, or using the transport of the department of agriculture for the emergency evacuation of sick patients.

A "whole-of-government approach", aiming for "health in all policies" follows a different logic[41,42]. It does not start from a specific health problem and look at how other sectors can contribute to solving them – as would be the case, for example, for tobacco-related disease. It starts by looking at the effects of agricultural, educational, environmental, fiscal, housing, transport and other policies on health. It then seeks to work with these other sectors to ensure that, while contributing to well-being and wealth, these policies also contribute to health[5].

Other sector's public policies, as well as private sector policies, can be important to health in two ways.

■ Some may lead to adverse consequences for health (Table 4.1). Often such adverse consequences are identified retrospectively, as in the case of the negative health effects of air pollution or industrial contamination. Yet, it is also often possible to foresee them or detect them at an early stage. Decision-makers in other sectors may be unaware of the consequences of the choices they are making, in which case engagement, with due consideration for the other sectors' goals and objectives, may then be the first step in minimizing the adverse health effects.

■ Public policies developed by other sectors – education, gender equality and social inclusion – may positively contribute to health in ways that these other sectors are equally unaware of. They may be further enhanced by more purposefully pursuing these positive health outcomes, as an integral part of the policy. For example, a gender equality policy, developed in its own right, may produce health benefits, often to a degree that the proponents of the policy underestimate. By collaborating to give more formal recognition to these outcomes, the gender equality policy itself is reinforced, and the synergies enhance the health outcomes. In that case, the objective of intersectoral collaboration is to reinforce the synergies.

Failing to collaborate with other sectors is not without its consequences. It affects the performance of health systems and, particularly, primary care. For example, Morocco's trachoma programme relied both on high levels of community mobilization and on effective collaboration with the ministries of education, interior and local affairs. That collaboration has been the key to the successful elimination of trachoma[43]. In contrast, the same country's tuberculosis control programme failed to link up with urban development and poverty reduction efforts and, as a result, its performance has been disappointing[44]. Both were administered by the same Ministry of Health, by staff with similar capacities working under similar resource constraints, but with different strategies.

Failing to collaborate with other sectors has another consequence, which is that avoidable ill-health is not avoided. In the NGagne Diaw quarter of Thiaroye-sur-Mer, Dakar, Senegal, people make a living from the informal recycling of lead batteries. This was of little concern to the authorities until an unexplained cluster of child deaths prompted an investigation. The area was found to be contaminated with lead, and the siblings and mothers of the dead children were found to have extremely high concentrations of lead in their blood. Now, major investments are required to deal with the health and social consequences and to decontaminate the affected area, including people's homes. Before the cluster of deaths occurred, the health sector had, unfortunately, not considered it a priority to work with other sectors to help to avoid this situation[45].

Where intersectoral collaboration is successful, the health benefits can be considerable, although deaths avoided are less readily noticed than lives lost. For example, pressure from civil society and professionals led to the development, in France, of a multi-pronged, high-profile strategy to improve road safety as a social and political issue that had to be confronted (and not primarily as a health sector issue). Various sectors worked together in a sustained effort, with high-level political endorsement, to reduce road-traffic accidents, with highly publicized monitoring of progress and a reduction in fatalities of up to 21% per year[46]. The health and health equity benefits of working towards health in all policies have become apparent in programmes such as "Healthy Cities and Municipalities", "Sustainable Cities", and "Cities Without Slums", with integrated approaches that range from engagement in budget hearings and social accountability mechanisms to data gathering and environmental intervention[47].

In contemporary societies, health tends to become fragmented into various sub-institutions dealing with particular aspects of health or health systems, while the capacity to assemble the various aspects of public policy that jointly determine health is underdeveloped. Even in the well-resourced context of, for example, the European Union, the institutional basis for doing this remains poorly developed[48]. Ministries of health have a vital role to play in creating such a basis, which is among the key strategies for making headway in tackling the socioeconomic determinants of ill-health[49].

Understanding the under-investment

Despite the benefits and low relative cost of better public policies, their potential remains largely underutilized across the world. One high-profile example is that only 5% of the world's population live in countries with comprehensive tobacco advertising, promotion and sponsorship bans, despite their proven efficacy in reducing health threats, which are projected to claim one billion lives this century[50].

The health sector's approach to improving public policies has been singularly unsystematic and guided by patchy evidence and muddled decision-making – not least because the health community has put so little effort into collating and communicating these facts. For all the progress that has been made in recent years, information on the effectiveness of interventions to redress, for example, health inequities is still hard to come by and, when it is available, it is confined to a privileged circle of concerned experts. A lack of information and evidence is, thus, one of the explanations for under-investment.

Box 4.3 How to make unpopular public policy decisions[51]

The Seventh Futures Forum of senior health executives organized by the World Health Organization's Regional Office for Europe in 2004 discussed the difficulties decision-makers can have in tackling unpopular policy decisions. A popular decision is usually one that results from broad public demand; an unpopular decision does not often respond to clearly expressed public expectations, but is made because the minister or the chief medical officer knows it is the right action to bring health gains and improve quality. Thus, a potentially unpopular decision should not seek popularity but, rather, efforts must be made to render it understandable and, therefore, acceptable. Making decisions more popular is not an academic exercise but one that deals with actual endorsement. When a decision is likely to be unpopular, participants in the Forum agreed that it is advisable for health executives to apply some of the following approaches.

Talk about health and quality improvement. Health is the core area of expertise and competence, and the explanations of how the decision will improve the quality of health and health services should therefore come first. Avoiding non-health arguments that are difficult to promote may be useful – for instance, in the case of hospital closures, it is much better to talk about improving quality of care than about containing costs.

Offer compensation. Explain what people will receive to balance what they will have to give up. Offer some gains in other sectors or in other services; work to make a win-win interpretation of the coming decision by balancing good and bad news.

Be strong on implementation. If health authorities are not ready to implement the decision, they should refrain from introducing it until they are ready to do so.

Be transparent. Explain who is taking the decision and the stakes of those involved and those who are affected. Enumerate all the stakeholders and whether they [are] involved negatively.

Avoid one-shot decisions. Design and propose the decisions as part of an overall plan or strategy.

Ensure good timing. Before making a decision, it is essential to take enough time to prepare and develop a good plan. When the plan is ready, the best choice may be to act quickly for implementation.

Involve all groups. Bring into the discussion both the disadvantaged groups and the ones who will benefit from the decision. Diversify the approach.

Do not expect mass-media support solely because the decision is the right one from the viewpoint of health gains. The mass media cannot be expected to be always neutral or positive; they may often be brought into the debate by the opponents of the decision. Be prepared to face problems with the press.

Be modest. Acceptability of the decision is more likely when decision-makers acknowledge in public that there is some uncertainty about the result and they commit openly to monitoring and evaluating the outcomes. This leaves the door open for adjustments during the process of implementation.

Be ready for quick changes. Sometimes the feelings of the public change quickly and what was perceived as opposition can turn into acceptance.

Be ready for crisis and unexpected side-effects. Certain groups of populations can be especially affected by a decision (such as general practitioners in the case of hospital closures). Public-health decision-makers have to cope with reactions that were not planned.

Stick to good evidence. Public acceptance may be low without being based on any objective grounds. Having good facts is a good way to shape the debate and avoid resistance.

Use examples from other countries. Decision-makers may look at what is being done elsewhere and explain why other countries deal with a problem differently; they can use such arguments to make decisions more acceptable in their own country.

Involve health professionals and, above all, *be courageous.*

The fact is, however, that even for well-informed political decision-makers, many public policy issues have a huge potential for unpopularity: whether it is reducing the number of hospital beds, imposing seatbelts, culling poultry or taxing alcohol, resistance is to be expected and controversy an everyday occurrence. Other decisions have so little visibility, e.g. measures that ensure a safe food production chain, that they offer little political mileage. Consensus on stern measures may be easy to obtain at a moment of crisis, but public opinion has a notoriously short attention span. Politicians often pay more attention to policies that produce benefits within electoral cycles of two to four years and, therefore, undervalue efforts where benefits, such as those of environmental protection or early child development, accrue over a time span of 20 to 40 years. If unpopularity is one intractable disincentive to political commitment, active opposition from well-resourced lobbies is another. An obvious example is the tobacco industry's efforts to limit tobacco control. Similar opposition is seen to the regulation of industrial waste and to the marketing of food to children. These obstacles to steering public policy are real and need to be dealt with in a systematic way (Box 4.3).

Compounding these disincentives to political commitment is the difficulty of coordinating operations across multiple institutions and sectors. Many countries have limited institutional capacity to do so and, very often, do not have enough capable professionals to cope with the work involved. Crisis management, short-term planning horizons, lack of understandable evidence, unclear intersectoral arrangements, vested interests and inadequate modes of governing the health sector reinforce the need for comprehensive policy reforms to realize the potential of public-health action. Fortunately, there are promising opportunities to build upon.

Opportunities for better public policies

Better information and evidence

Although there are strong indications that the potential gains from better public policies are enormous, the evidence base on their outcomes and on their cost-effectiveness is surprisingly weak[52]. We know much about the relationship between certain behaviours – smoking, diet, exercise, etc. – and health outcomes, but much less about how to effect behavioural change in a systematic and sustainable way at population levels. Even in well-resourced contexts, the obstacles are many: the time-scale in achieving outcomes; the complexity of multifactorial disease causation and intervention effects; the lack of data; the methodological problems, including the difficulties in applying the well-accepted criteria used in the evaluation of clinical methods; and the different perspectives of the multiple stakeholders involved. Infectious disease surveillance is improving, but information on chronic diseases and their determinants or on health inequities is patchy and often lacks systematic focus. Even the elementary foundations for work on population health and the collection of statistics on births and deaths or diseases are deficient in many countries (Box 4.4)[53].

Over the last 30 years, however, there has been a quantum leap in the production of evidence for clinical medicine through collaborative efforts such as the Cochrane Collaboration and the International Clinical Epidemiology Network[56,57]. A similar advance is possible in the production of evidence on public policies, although such efforts are still too tentative compared to the enormous resources available for research in other areas of health, e.g. diagnostic and therapeutic medical technologies. There are, however, signs of progress in the increasing use of systematic reviews by policy-makers[58,59].

Two tracks offer potential for significantly strengthening the knowledge base.

■ Speeding up the organization of systematic reviews of critical interventions and their economic evaluation. One way of doing this is by expanding the remit of existing health technology assessment agencies to include the assessment of public-health interventions and delivery modes, since this would make use of existing institutional capacities with ring-fenced resources. The emerging collaborative networks, such as the Campbell Collaboration[60], can play a catalyzing role, exploiting

---

Box 4.4 The scandal of invisibility: where births and deaths are not counted

Civil registration is both a product of economic and social development, and a condition for modernization. There has been little improvement in coverage of vital registration (official recording of births and deaths) over recent decades (see Figure 4.3). Almost 40% (48 million) of 128 million global births each year go uncounted because of the lack of civil[53] registration systems. The situation is even worse for deaths registration. Globally, two thirds (38 million) of 57 million annual deaths are not registered. WHO receives reliable cause-of-death statistics from only 31 of its 193 Member States.

International efforts to improve vital statistics infrastructure in developing countries have been too limited in size and scope[54]. Neither, the global health community nor the countries have given the development of health statistics and civil registration systems the same priority

as health interventions. Within the UN system, civil registration development has no identifiable home. There are no coordination mechanisms to tackle the problem and respond to requests for technical support for mobilizing the necessary financial and technical resources. Establishing the infrastructure of civil registration systems to ensure all births and deaths are counted requires collaboration between different partners in different sectors. It needs sustained advocacy, the nurturing of public trust, supportive legal frameworks, incentives, financial support, human resources and modernized data management systems[55]. Where it functions well, vital statistics provide basic information for priority setting. The lack of progress in the registration of births and deaths is a major concern for the design and implementation of PHC reforms.

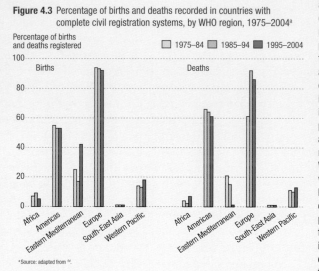

Figure 4.3 Percentage of births and deaths recorded in countries with complete civil registration systems, by WHO region, 1975–2004[a]

Percentage of births and deaths registered

☐ 1975–84 ☐ 1985–94 ■ 1995–2004

[a] Source: adapted from[54].

---

the comparative advantage of scale efficiency and international comparisons.

■ Accelerating the documentation and assessment of whole-of-government approaches using techniques that build on the initial experience with "health impact assessment" or "health equity impact assessment" tools[61,62,63]. Although these tools are still in development, there is growing demand from local to supra-national policy-makers for such analyses (Box 4.5). Evidence of their utility in influencing public policies is building up[64,65,66], and they constitute a strategic way of organizing more thoughtful cross-sector discussions. That in itself is an inroad into one of the more intractable aspects of the use of the available evidence base: the clear need for more systematic communication on the potential health gains to be derived from better public policies. Decision-makers, particularly in other sectors, are insufficiently aware of the

health consequences of their policies, and of the potential benefits that could be derived from them. Communication beyond the realm of the specialist is as important as the production of evidence and requires far more effective approaches to the dissemination of evidence among policy-makers[67]. Framing population health evidence in terms of the health impact of policies, rather than in the classical modes of communication among health specialists, has the potential to change radically the type and quality of policy dialogue.

A changing institutional landscape

Along with lack of evidence, the area where new opportunities are appearing is in the institutional capacity for developing public policies that are aligned with PHC goals. Despite the reluctance, including from donors, to commit substantial funds to National Institutes of Public Health (NIPHs)[69], policy-makers rely heavily on them or

---

Box 4.5 European Union impact assessment guidelines[68]

European Union guidelines suggest that the answers to the following questions can form the basis of an assessment of the impact of proposed public-health interventions.

Public health and safety

Does the proposed option:

- affect the health and safety of individuals or populations, including life expectancy, mortality and morbidity through impacts on the socioeconomic environment, e.g. working environment, income, education, occupation or nutrition?
- increase or decrease the likelihood of bioterrorism?
- increase or decrease the likelihood of health risks attributable to substances that are harmful to the natural environment?
- affect health because of changes in the amount of noise or air, water or soil quality in populated areas?
- affect health because of changes in energy use or waste disposal?
- affect lifestyle-related determinants of health such as the consumption of tobacco or alcohol, or physical activity?
- produce specific effects on particular risk groups (determined by age, sex, disability, social group, mobility, region, etc.)?

Access to and effects on social protection, health and educational systems

Does the proposed option:

- have an impact on services in terms of their quality and access to them?
- have an effect on the education and mobility of workers (health, education, etc.)?
- affect the access of individuals to public or private education or vocational and continuing training?
- affect the cross-border provision of services, referrals across borders and cooperation in border regions?
- affect the financing and organization of and access to social, health and education systems (including vocational training)?
- affect universities and academic freedom or self-governance?

---

on their functional equivalents. In many countries, NIPHs have been the primary repositories of independent technical expertise for public health, but also, more broadly, for public policies. Some have a prestigious track record: the Fiocruz in Brazil, the Instituto de Medicina Tropical "Pedro Kouri" in Cuba, Kansanterveyslaitos in Finland, the Centers for Disease Control and Prevention in the United States, or the National Institute of Hygiene and Epidemiology in Viet Nam. They testify to the importance that countries accord to being able to rely on such capacity[69]. Increasingly, however, this capacity is unable to cope with the multiple new demands for public policies to protect or promote health. This is leaving traditional national and global institutes of public health with an oversized, under-funded mandate, which poses problems of dispersion and difficulties in assembling the critical mass of diversified and specialized expertise (Figure 4.4).

In the meantime, the institutional landscape is changing as the capacity for public policy support is being spread over a multitude of national and supra-national institutions. The number of loci of expertise, often specialized in some aspect of public policy, has increased considerably,

spanning a broad range of institutional forms including: research centres, foundations, academic units, independent consortia and think tanks, projects, technical agencies and assorted initiatives. Malaysia's Health Promotion Foundation Board, New Zealand's Alcohol Advisory

Figure 4.4 Essential public-health functions that 30 national public-health institutions view as being part of their portfolio[69]

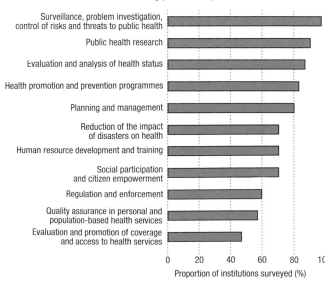

Council and Estonia's Health Promotion Commission show that funding channels have diversified and may include research grants and contracts, government subsidies, endowments, or hypothecated taxes on tobacco and alcohol sales. This results in a more complex and diffuse, but also much richer, network of expertise.

There are important scale efficiencies to be obtained from cross-border collaboration on a variety of public policy issues. For example, the International Association of National Public Health Institutes (IANPHI) helps countries to set up strategies for institutional capacity development[70]. In this context, institution building will have to establish careful strategies for specialization and complementarity, paying attention to the challenge of leadership and coordination.

At the same time, this offers perspectives for transforming the production of the highly diverse and specialized workforce that better public policies require. Schools of public health, community medicine and community nursing have traditionally been the primary institutional reservoirs for generating that workforce. However, they produce too few professionals who are too often focused on disease control and classical epidemiology, and are usually ill-prepared for a career of flexibility, continuous learning and coordinated leadership.

The multi-centric institutional development provides opportunities for a fundamental rethink of curricula and of the institutional settings of pre-service education, with on-the-job training in close contact with the institutions where the expertise is located and developed[71]. There are promising signs of renewal in this regard in the WHO South-East Asian Region (SEARO) that should be drawn upon to stimulate similar thinking and action elsewhere[27]. The increasing cross-border exchange of experience and expertise, combined with a global interest in improving public policy-making capacity, is creating new opportunities – not just in order to prepare professionals in more adequate numbers but, above all, professionals with a broader outlook and who are better prepared to address complex public heath challenges of the future.

Equitable and efficient global health action

In many countries, responsibilities for health and social services are being delegated to local levels. At the same time, financial, trade, industrial and agricultural policies are shifting to international level: health outcomes have to be obtained locally, while health determinants are being influenced at international level. Countries increasingly align their public policies with those of a globalized world. This presents both opportunities and risks.

In adjusting to globalization, fragmented policy competencies in national governance systems are finding convergence. Various ministries, including health, agriculture, finance, trade and foreign affairs are now exploring together how they can best inform pre-negotiation trade positions, provide input during negotiations, and weigh the costs and benefits of alternative policy options on health, the economy and the future of their people. This growing global health "interdependence" is accompanied by a mushrooming of activities expressed at the global level. The challenge is, therefore, to ensure that emerging networks of governance are adequately inclusive of all actors and sectors, responsive to local needs and demands, accountable, and oriented towards social justice[72]. The recent emergence of a global food crisis provides further legitimacy to an input from the health sector into the evolving global response. Gradually, a space is opening for the consideration of health in the trade agreements negotiated through the World Trade Organization (WTO). Although implementation has proved problematic, the flexibilities agreed at Doha for provision in the Agreement on Trade-Related Aspects of Intellectual Property Rights (TRIPS)[73] of compulsory licencing of pharmaceuticals are examples of emerging global policies to protect health.

There is a growing demand for global norms and standards as health threats are being shifted from areas where safety measures are being tightened to places where they barely exist. Assembling the required expertise and processes is complex and expensive. Increasingly, countries are relying on global mechanisms and collaboration[74]. This trend started over 40 years ago with the creation of the Codex Alimentarius Commission in 1963 by the Food and Agriculture Organization (FAO) and the WHO to coordinate international food standards and consumer protection. Another long-standing example is the International Programme on Chemical Safety, established in 1980 as a joint programme of the WHO, the International Labour Organization (ILO) and the United Nations Environment Programme (UNEP). In the European Union, the construction of health protection standards is shared between agencies and applied across Europe. Given the expense and complexity of drug safety monitoring, many countries adapt and use the standards of the United States Food and Drug Administration (FDA). WHO sets global standards for tolerable levels of many

contaminants. In the meantime, countries must either undertake these processes themselves or ensure access to standards from other countries or international agencies, adapted to their own context.

The imperative for global public-health action, thus, places further demands on the capacity and strength of health leadership to respond to the need to protect the health of their communities. Local action needs to be accompanied by the coordination of different stakeholders and sectors within countries. It also needs to manage global health challenges through global collaboration and negotiation. As the next chapter shows, this is a key responsibility of the state.

References

1. Sen A. *Development as freedom*. Oxford, Oxford University Press, 1999.
2. Fegan GW et al. Effect of expanded insecticide-treated bednet coverage on child survival in rural Kenya: a longitudinal study. *Lancet*, 2007, 370:1035–1039.
3. Liu Y. China's public health-care system: facing the challenges. *Bulletin of the World Health Organization*, 2004, 82:532–538.
4. Kaufman JA. China's heath care system and avian influenza preparedness. *Journal of Infectious Diseases*, 2008, 197(Suppl. 1):S7–S13.
5. Ståhl T et al, eds. *Health in all policies: prospects and potentials*. Helsinki, Ministry of Social Affairs and Health, 2006.
6. Berer M. National laws and unsafe abortion: the parameters of change. Reproductive Health Matters, 2004, 12:1–8.
7. Grimes DA et al. Unsafe abortion: the preventable pandemic. *Lancet*, 2006, 368:1908–1919.
8. Sommer A, Mosley WH. East Bengal cyclone of November 1970: epidemiological approach to disaster assessment. *Lancet*, 1972, 1:1029–1036.
9. Bern C et al. Risk factors for mortality in the Bangladesh cyclone of 1991. *Bulletin of the World Health Organization*, 1993, 71:73–78.
10. Chowdhury AM. Personal communication, 2008.
11. Asaria P et al. Chronic disease prevention: health effects and financial costs of strategies to reduce salt intake and control tobacco use. *Lancet*, 2007, 370:2044–2053.
12. *World abortion policies 2007*. New York NY, United Nations, Department of Economic and Social Affairs, Population Division, 2007 (ST/ESA/SER.A/264, Wallchart).
13. *Unsafe abortion. Global and regional estimates of the incidence of unsafe abortion and associated mortality in 2003*, 5th ed. Geneva, World Health Organization, 2007.
14. *Maternal health and early childhood development in Cuba*. Ottawa, Committee on Social Affairs, Science and Technology, 2007 (Second Report of the Subcommittee on Population Health of the Standing Senate).
15. Evans RG. Thomas McKeown, meet Fidel Castro: physicians, population health and the Cuban paradox. *Healthcare Policy*, 2008, 3:21–32.
16. Spiegel JM, Yassi A. Lessons from the margins of globalization: appreciating the Cuban health paradox. *Journal of Public Health Policy*, 2004, 25:85–110.
17. *The World Health Report – Health systems: improving performance*. Geneva, World Health Organization, 2000.
18. *Everybody's business – strengthening health systems to improve health outcomes*. Geneva, World Health Organization, Health Systems Services, 2007.
19. Hogerzeil HV. The concept of essential medicines: lessons for rich countries. *BMJ*, 2004, 329:1169–1172.
20. *Measuring medicine prices, availability, affordability and price components*, 2nd ed. Geneva, Health Action International and World Health Organization, 2008 (http://www.haiweb.org/medicineprices/, accessed 20 August 2008).
21. Black RE, Morris SS, Bryce J. Where and why are 10 million children dying every year? *Lancet*, 2003, 361:2226–2234.
22. *Supply annual report 2007*. Copenhagen, United Nations Children's Fund Supply Division, 2008.
23. Tambini G et al. Regional immunization programs as a model for strengthening cooperation among nations. *Revista panamericana de salud pública*, 2006, 20:54–59.
24. EPI Revolving Fund: quality vaccines at low cost. *EPI Newsletter*, 1997, 19:6–7.
25. Matiru R, Ryan T. The global drug facility: a unique, holistic and pioneering approach to drug procurement and management. *Bulletin of the World Health Organization*, 2007, 85:348–353.
26. *Annual Report*. Wellington, Pharmaceutical Management Agency, 2007.
27. *The World Health Report 2006 - Working together for health*. Geneva, World Health Organization, 2006.
28. Victora CG et al. Achieving universal coverage with health interventions. *Lancet*, 2004, 364:1555–1556.
29. Freitas do Amaral JJ et al. Multi-country evaluation of IMCI, Brazil study. Ceará, Federal University of Ceará, ND.
30. Sontag S. *AIDS and its metaphors*. New York, NY, Farrar, Straus & Giroux, 1988.
31. Mann JM et al, eds. *Health and human rights: a reader*. New York NY, Routledge, 1999.
32. Friedman S, Mottiar S. A rewarding engagement? The treatment action campaign and the politics of HIV/AIDS. *Politics and Society*, 2005, 33:511–565.
33. Ottawa Charter for Health Promotion. In: *First International Conference on Health Promotion, Ottawa, 21 November 1986*. Geneva, World Health Organization, Department of Human Resources for Health, 1986 (WHO/HPR/HEP/95.1; http://www.who.int/hpr/NPH/docs/ottawa_charter_hp.pdf, accessed 2 July 2008).
34. Ezzati M et al. Comparative risk assessment collaborating group. Estimates of global and regional potential health gains from reducing multiple major risk factors. *Lancet*, 2003, 362:271–280..
35. Friel S, Chopra M, Satcher D. Unequal weight: equity oriented policy responses to the global obesity epidemic. *BMJ*, 2007, 335:1241–1243.
36. Satcher D, Higginbotham EJ. The public health approach to eliminating disparities in health. *American Journal of Public Health*, 2008, 98:400–403.

37. Commission on Social Determinants of Health. *Closing the gap in a generation: health equity through action on the social determinants of health. Final report.* Geneva, World Health Organization, 2008.

38. *The World Health Report 2007 – A safer future: global public health security in the 21st century.* Geneva, World Health Organization, 2007

39. Satterthwaite D. In pursuit of a healthy urban environment. In: Marcotullkio PJ, McGranahan G, eds. *Scaling urban environmental challenges: from local to global and back.* London, Earthscan, 2007.

40. Taylor CE, Taylor HG. Scaling up community-based primary health care. In: Rohde J, Wyon J, eds. *Community-based health care: lessons from Bangladesh to Boston.* Boston, Management Sciences for Health, 2002.

41. WHO/Public Health Agency Canada Collaborative Project. *Improving health equity through intersectoral action.* Geneva, World Health Organization, 2008 (in press).

42. Puska P. Health in all policies. *European Journal of Public Health*, 2007, 17:328.

43. Chami Y, Hammou J, Mahjour J. Lessons from the Moroccan national trachoma control programme. *Community Eye Health*, 2004, 17:59.

44. Dye C et al. The decline of tuberculosis epidemics under chemotherapy: a case study in Morocco. *International Journal of Tuberculosis and Lung Disease*, 2007, 11:1225–1231.

45. *Senegal: outbreak of lead intoxication in Thiaroye sur Mer 20 June 2008.* Geneva, World Health Organization, 2008 (http://www.who.int/environmental_health_emergencies/events/Senegal2008/en/index.html, accessed 21 July 2008).

46. Muhlrad N. *Road safety management in France: political leadership as a path to sustainable progress.* Paper presented at: Gambit 2004 Road Safety Conference, Gdansk, April 2004.

47. *Our cities, our health, our future: acting on social determinants for health equity in urban settings.* Geneva, World Health Organization, 2007.

48. Koivusalo M. Moving health higher up the European agenda. In: Ståhl T et al, eds. *Health in all policies: prospects and potentials.* Helsinki, Ministry of Social Affairs and Health, 2006:21–40.

49. Gilson L et al. *Challenging health inequity through health systems.* Geneva, World Health Organization, 2007.

50. *WHO report on the global tobacco epidemic, 2008: the MPOWER package.* Geneva, World Health Organization, 2008.

51. Anaudova A. *Seventh Futures Forum on Unpopular Decisions in Public Health.* Copenhagen, World Health Organization Regional Office for Europe, 2005.

52. Allin S et al. *Making decisions on public health: a review of eight countries.* Geneva, World Health Organization, European Observatory on Health Systems and Policies, 2004.

53. Setel PW et al. on behalf of the Monitoring of Vital Events (MoVE) writing group. A scandal of invisibility: making everyone count by counting everyone. *Lancet,* 2007 (published online: DOI: 10.1016/S0140-6736(07)61307-5).

54. Mahapatra P et al. on behalf of the Monitoring of Vital Events (MoVE) writing group. Civil registration systems and vital statistics: successes and missed opportunities. *Lancet,* 2007 (published online: DOI: 10.1016/S0140-6736(07)61308-7).

55. AbouZahr C et al. on behalf of the Monitoring of Vital Events (MoVE) writing group. The way forward. *Lancet,* 2007 (published online: DOI: 10.1016/S0140-6736(07)61310-5).

56. Volmink J et al. AM. Research synthesis and dissemination as a bridge to knowledge management: the Cochrane Collaboration. *Bulletin of the World Health Organization,* 2004, 82:778–783.

57. Halstead SB, Tugwell P, Bennett K. The International Clinical Epidemiology Network (INCLEN): a progress report. *Journal of Clinical Epidemiology*, 1991, 44:579–589.

58. Waters E et al. Cochrane Collaboration. Evaluating the effectiveness of public health interventions: the role and activities of the Cochrane Collaboration. *Journal of Epidemiology and Community Health*, 2006, 60:285–289.

59. Sweet M, Moynihan R. *Improving population health: the uses of systematic reviews.* New York NY, Milbank Memorial Fund, 2007.

60. Davies P, Boruch R. The Campbell Collaboration does for public policy what Cochrane does for health. *BMJ*, 2001, 323:294–295.

61. *An idea whose time has come: New opportunities for HIA in New Zealand public policy and planning.* Wellington, Public Health Advisory Committee, 2007.

62. Harris P et al. *Health impact assessment: a practical guide.* Sydney, University of New South Wales, 2007.

63. Wismar M et al. Implementing and institutionalizing health impact assessment in Europe. In: Ståhl T et al, eds. *Health in all policies: prospects and potentials.* Helsinki, Ministry of Social Affairs and Health, 2006.

64. Blau J et al. The use of health impact assessment across Europe. In: Ståhl T et al, eds. *Health in all policies: prospects and potentials.* Helsinki, Ministry of Social Affairs and Health, 2006.

65. Dannenberg AL et al. Use of health impact assessment in the US: 27 case studies, 1999–2007. *American Journal of Preventive Medicine*, 2008, 34:241–256.

66. Wismar M et al. eds. *The effectiveness of health impact assessment: scope and limitations of supporting decision-making in Europe.* Geneva, World Health Organization, 2007.

67. Jewell CJ, Bero LA. Developing good taste in evidence: facilitators of and hindrances to evidence-informed health policymaking in state government. *The Milbank Quarterly*, 2008, 86:177–208.

68. *Communication from the Commission on Better Regulation for Growth and Jobs in the European Union.* Brussels, European Commission, 2005 (COM (2005) 97 final).

69. Binder S et al. National public health institutes: contributing to the public good. *Journal of Public Health Policy*, 2008, 29:3–21.

70. *Framework for the creation and development of national public health institutes.* Helsinki, International Association of National Public Health Institutes, 2007.

71. Khaleghian P, Das Gupta M. *Public management and the essential public health functions.* Washington DC, The World Bank, 2004 (World Bank Policy Research Working Paper 3220).

72. Kickbusch I. A new agenda for health. *Perspectives in Health*, 2004, 9:8–13.

73. *World Trade Organization Declaration on the TRIPS Agreement and Public Health. Ministerial Conference, 4th Session, Doha, 9–14 November 2001.* 2001 (WT/MIN(01)/DEC/2).

74. Wilk EA van der et al. *Learning from our neighbours – cross-national inspiration for Dutch public health polices: smoking, alcohol, overweight, depression, health inequalities, youth screening.* Bilthoven, National Institute for Public Health and the Environment, 2008 (RIVM Rapport 270626001; http://www.rivm.nl/bibliotheek/rapporten/270626001.pdf, accessed 30 July 2008).

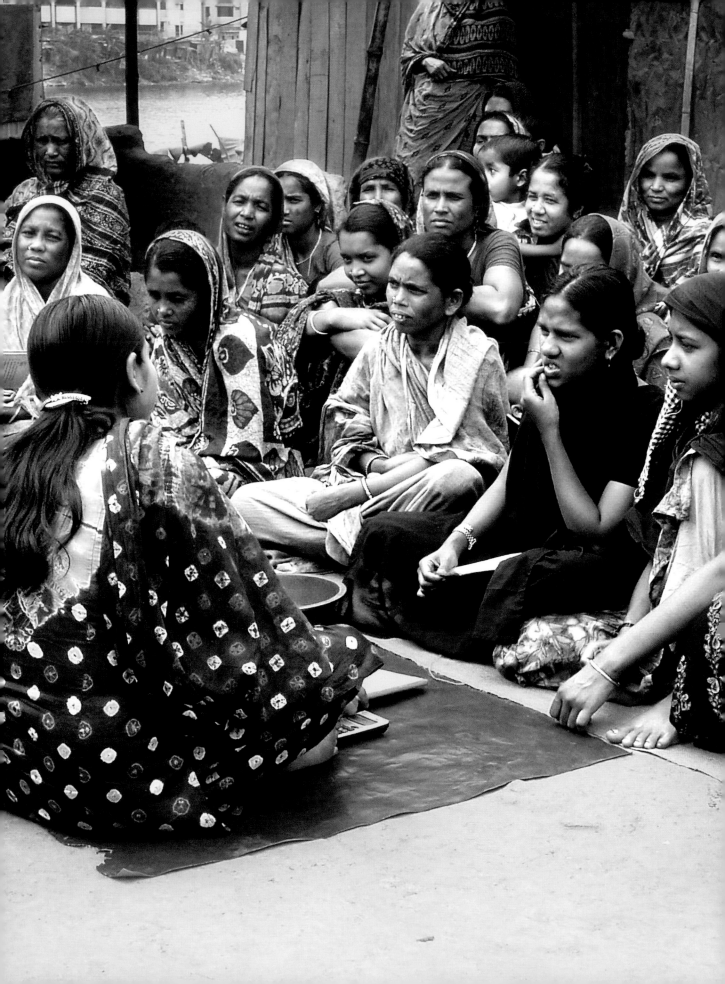

Leadership and
effective government

◆◆ *The preceding chapters have described how health systems can be transformed to deliver better health in ways that people value: equitably, people-centred, and with the knowledge that health authorities administer public-health functions to secure the well-being of all communities. These PHC reforms demand new forms of leadership for health. This chapter begins by clarifying why the public sector needs to have a strong role in leading and steering public health care reforms, and emphasizes the fact that this function should be exercised through collaborative models of policy dialogue with multiple stakeholders, because this is what people expect and because it is the most effective. It then considers strategies to improve the effectiveness of reform efforts and the management of the political processes that condition them.*

Chapter 5

Governments as brokers for PHC reform

Mediating the social contract for health

The ultimate responsibility for shaping national health systems lies with governments. Shaping does not suggest that governments should – or even could – reform the entire health sector on their own. Many different groups have a role to play: national politicians and local governments, the health professions, the scientific community, the private sector and civil society organizations, as well as the global health community. Nevertheless, the responsibility for health that is entrusted to government agencies is unique and is rooted in principled politics as well as in widely held expectations[1].

Politically, the legitimacy of governments and their popular support depends on their ability to protect their citizens and play a redistributive role. The governance of health is among the core public policy instruments for institutionalized protection and redistribution. In modern states, governments are expected to protect health, to guarantee access to health care and to safeguard people from the impoverishment that illness can bring. These responsibilities were progressively extended, incorporating the correction of market failures that characterize the health sector[2]. Since the beginning of the 20th century, health protection and health care have progressively been incorporated as goods that are guaranteed by governments and are central to the social contract between the state and its citizens. The importance of health systems as a key element of the social contract in modernizing societies is most acutely evident during reconstruction after periods of war or disaster: rebuilding health services counts among the first tangible signs that society is returning to normal[3].

The legitimacy of state intervention is not only based on social and political considerations. There are also key economic actors – the medical equipment industry, the pharmaceutical industry and the professions – with an interest in governments taking responsibility for health to ensure a viable health market: a costly modern health economy cannot be sustained without risk

sharing and pooling of resources. Indeed, those countries that spend the most on health are also those countries with the largest public financing of the health sector (Figure 5.1).

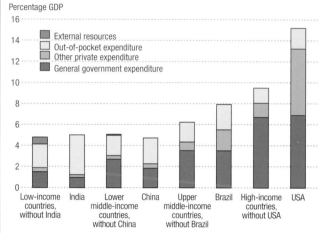

Figure 5.1 Percentage of GDP used for health, 2005[4]

Percentage GDP

Legend:
- External resources
- Out-of-pocket expenditure
- Other private expenditure
- General government expenditure

Categories: Low-income countries, without India; India; Lower middle-income countries, without China; China; Upper middle-income countries, without Brazil; Brazil; High-income countries, without USA; USA

Even in the United States, its exceptionalism stems not from lower public expenditure – at 6.9% of GDP it is no lower than the high-income countries average of 6.7% – but from its singularly high additional private expenditure. The persistent under-performance of the United States health sector across domains of health outcomes, quality, access, efficiency and equity[5], explains opinion polls that show increasing consensus of the notion of government intervention to secure more equitable access to essential health care[6,7].

A more effective public sector stewardship of the health sector is, thus, justified on the grounds of greater efficiency and equity. This crucial stewardship role is often misinterpreted as a mandate for centralized planning and complete administrative control of the health sector. While some types of health challenges, e.g. public-health emergencies or disease eradication, may require authoritative command-and-control management, effective stewardship increasingly relies on "mediation" to address current and future complex health challenges. The interests of public authorities, the health sector and the public are closely intertwined. Over the years, this has made all the institutions of medical care, such as training, accreditation, payment, hospitals, entitlements, etc., the object of intensive bargaining on how broadly to define the welfare state and the collective goods that go with it[8,9]. This means that public and quasi-public institutions have to mediate the social contract between institutions of medicine, health and society[10]. In high-income countries today, the health-care system and the state appear indissolubly bound together. In low- and middle-income countries, the state has often had a more visible role, but paradoxically, one that was less effective in steering the health sector, particularly when, during the 1980s and 1990s, some countries of them became severely tested by conflicts and economic recession. This resulted in their health systems being drawn in directions quite different from the goals and values pursued by the PHC movement.

Disengagement and its consequences

In many socialist and post-socialist countries undergoing economic restructuring, the state has withdrawn abruptly from its previously predominant role in health. China's deregulation of the health sector in the 1980s, and the subsequent steep increases in reliance on out-of-pocket spending, is a case in point and a warning to the rest of the world[11]. A spectacular deterioration of health-care provision and social protection, particularly in rural areas, led to a marked slowdown in the increase in life expectancy[11,12]. This caused China to re-examine its policies and reassert the Government's leadership role – a re-examination that is far from over (Box 5.1)[13].

A similar scenario of disengagement was observed in many of the countries of central and eastern Europe and the Commonwealth of Independent States (CEE-CIS). In the early 1990s, public expenditure on health declined to levels that made administering a basic system virtually impossible. This contributed to a major decline in life expectancy[17]. Catastrophic health spending became a major cause of poverty[18]. More recently, funding levels have stabilized or even increased, but significant improvements in health outcomes have not followed and socioeconomic inequalities in health and health-care access are rising. Evidence and trends related to these rises, as well as increases in informal payment mechanisms

for health care, indicate that re-engagement is still insufficient.

Elsewhere, but most spectacularly in low-income countries and fragile states, the absence or withdrawal of the state from its responsibilities for health reflects broader conditions of economic stagnation, political and social crisis and poor governance[19]. In such conditions, public leadership has often become dysfunctional and de-institutionalized[20], a weakness that is compounded by a lack of financial leverage to steer the health sector. Global development policies have often added to the difficulties governments face in assuming their responsibilities, for at least two reasons.

- The global development agenda of the 1980s and 1990s was dominated by concern for the problems created by too much state involvement[21]. The structural adjustment and downsizing recipes of these decades still constrain the reconstruction of leadership capacity today. Public financing in the poorest countries became unpredictable, making medium-term commitments to the growth of the health sector difficult or impossible. Health planning based on needs became the exception rather than the rule, since key fiscal decisions were taken with little understanding of the potential consequences for the health sector and health ministries were unable to make an effective case for prioritizing budget increases[22].

- For decades, the international community's health agenda – including that of WHO – has been structured around diseases and interventions rather than around the broader challenges being faced by health systems. While this agenda has certainly contributed to a better appreciation of the burden of disease affecting poor countries, it has also profoundly influenced the structure of governmental and quasi-governmental institutions in low- and middle-income countries. The resulting fragmentation of the governance of the health sector has diverted attention from important issues, such as the organization of primary care, the control of the commercialization of the health sector and human resources for health crises.

The untoward consequences of this trend are most marked in aid-dependent countries because it has shaped the way funds are channelled[23]. The disproportionate investment in a limited number of disease programmes considered as global priorities in countries that are dependent on external support has diverted the limited energies of ministries of health away from their primary role as mediator in the comprehensive planning of primary care and the public's health.

Box 5.1 From withdrawal to re-engagement in China

During the 1980s and 1990s, reduced Government engagement in the health sector exposed increasing numbers of Chinese households to catastrophic expenditures for health care. As a result, millions of families in both rural and urban areas found themselves unable to meet the costs and were effectively excluded from health care. In cities, the Government Insurance Scheme (GIS) and Labour Insurance Scheme (LIS) had previously covered more than half of the population with either full or partial health insurance. However, the structural weaknesses of these schemes reached critical levels under the impact of accelerating economic change in the 1990s. The percentage of China's urban population not covered by any health insurance or health plan rose from 27.3% in 1993 to 44.1% in 1998[14]. By the end of the century, out-of-pocket payments made up more than 60% of health expenditure. This crisis spurred efforts to invert the trend: pooling and pre-payment schemes were bolstered in 1998 with the introduction of Basic Medical Insurance (BMI) for urban employees.

Financed through compulsory contributions from workers and employers, the BMI aims to replace the old GIS and LIS systems. The BMI has aimed for breadth of coverage with a relatively modest depth of benefits, linked to flexibility that can enable the development of different types of packages according to local needs in the participating municipalities. Structurally, the BMI fund is divided into two parts: individual savings accounts and social pooling funds. Generally speaking, the financial contribution from an employee's salary or wages goes to his or her individual savings account, while the employer's contribution is split between the individual savings accounts and the social pooling fund, applying different percentages according to the age group of employees.

Financial resources under the new BMI are pooled at municipal or city level, instead of by individual enterprises, which significantly strengthens the capacity for risk sharing. Each municipal government has developed its own regulations on the use of the resources of individual savings accounts and social pooling funds (the two structural parts of the system). The individual savings accounts cover outpatient services, while the social pooling fund is meant to cover inpatient expenditures[14].

Significant difficulties with the BMI model remain to be ironed out, in particular as regards equity. For example, studies indicate that, in urban areas, better-off populations have been quicker to benefit from the provisions of the BMI than households with very low incomes, while informal sector workers remain on the margins of the scheme. Nonetheless, the BMI has made progress in expanding health insurance coverage and access to services among China's urban population, and is instrumental in reversing the deleterious trends of the 1980s and 1990s and, at the same time, assigning a new, intermediary role to government institutions.

Figure 5.2 Health expenditure in China: withdrawal of the State in the 1980s and 1990s and recent re-engagement

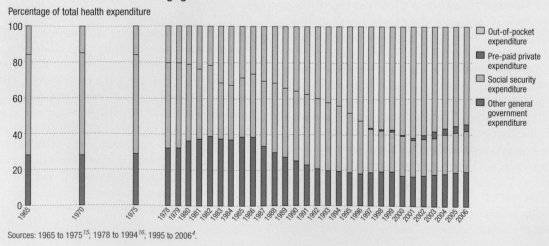

Percentage of total health expenditure

Sources: 1965 to 1975[15]; 1978 to 1994[16]; 1995 to 2006[4].

As a result, multiple, fragmented funding streams and segmented service delivery are leading to duplication, inefficiencies and counterproductive competition for resources between different programmes. Consequently, the massive mobilization of global solidarity has not been able to offset a growing estrangement between country needs and global support, and between people's expectations for decent care and the priorities set by their health-sector managers. Moreover, the growth in aid-flow mechanisms and new implementing institutions has further heightened the degree of complexity faced by weak government bureaucracies in donor-dependent countries, increasing transaction costs for those countries that can least afford them[24]. So much effort is required to respond to international partners' short-term agendas that little energy is left to deal with the multiple domestic stakeholders – professions, civil society organizations, politicians, and others – where, in the long run, leadership matters most. As advocates have rightly argued in recent years, better inter-donor coordination is not going to solve this problem on its own: there is also an urgent need for reinvestment in governance capacity.

Participation and negotiation

The necessary reinvestment in governmental or quasi-governmental institutions cannot mean a return to command-and-control health governance. Health systems are too complex: the domains of the modern state and civil society are interconnected, with constantly shifting boundaries[25]. Professions play a major role in how health is governed[26], while, as mentioned in Chapter 2, social movements and quasi-governmental autonomous institutions have become complex and influential political actors[27]. Patients, professions, commercial interests and other groups are organizing themselves in order to improve their negotiating position and to protect their interests. Ministries of health are, also, far from homogenous: individuals and programmes compete for influence and resources, adding to the complexity of promoting change. Effective mediation in health must replace overly simplistic management models of the past and embrace new mechanisms

for multi-stakeholder policy dialogue to work out the strategic orientations for PHC reforms[28].

At the core of policy dialogue is the participation of the key stakeholders. As countries modernize, their citizens attribute more value to social accountability and participation. Throughout the world, increasing prosperity, intellectual skills and social connectivity are associated with people's rising aspiration to have more say[29] in what happens at their workplaces and in their communities – hence the importance of people-centredness and community participation – and in important government decisions that affect their lives – hence the importance of involving civil society in the social debate on health policies[30].

Another reason that policy dialogue is so important is that PHC reforms require a broad policy dialogue to put the expectations of various stakeholders in perspective, to weigh up need, demand and future challenges, and to resolve the inevitable confrontations such reforms imply[31]. Health authorities and ministries of health, which have a primary role, have to bring together the decision-making power of the political authorities, the rationality of the scientific community, the commitment of the professionals, and the values and resources of civil society[32]. This is a process that requires time and effort (Box 5.2). It would be an illusion to expect PHC policy formation to be wholly consensual, as there are too many conflicting interests. However, experience shows that the legitimacy of policy choices depends less on total consensus than on procedural fairness and transparency[33,34,35].

Without a structured, participatory policy dialogue, policy choices are vulnerable to appropriation by interest groups, changes in political personnel or donor fickleness. Without a social consensus, it is also much more difficult to engage effectively with stakeholders whose interests diverge from the options taken by PHC reforms, including other sectors that compete for society's resources; for the "medico-industrial complex"[36], for whom PHC reform may imply a realignment of their industrial strategy and for vested interests, such as those of the tobacco or alcohol industries, where effective PHC reform constitutes a direct threat.

Box 5.2 Steering national directions with the help of policy dialogue: experience from three countries

In Canada, a Commission examining the future of health care drew on inputs from focus group discussions and public hearings. Diverse stakeholders and groups of the public made clear the value placed by Canadians on equitable access to high-quality care, based on need and regardless of ability to pay. At the same time, the Commission had to ensure that this debate would be fed by evidence from top policy experts on the realities of the country's health system. Of critical importance was the evidence that public financing of health care not only achieves goals of equity, but also those of efficiency, in view of the higher administrative costs associated with private financing. The discussion on values and the relevant evidence were then brought together in a policy report in 2002 that set out the direction for a responsive, sustainable and publicly funded PHC system, considered to be "the highest expression of Canadians caring for one another"[37]. The strong uptake by policy-makers of the Commission's recommendations reflects the robustness of the evidence-informed analysis and public engagement.

In Brazil, the first seven *Conferências Nacionais de Saúde,* the platform for national policy dialogue in the health sector between 1941 and 1977, had a distinctly top-down and public-sector-only flavour, with a classic progression from national plans to programmes and extension of the network of basic health services. The watershed came with the 8th conference in 1980: the number of participants increased from a few hundred to 4000, from a wide range of constituencies. This and subsequent *conferências* pursued agendas that were driven far more than before by values of health democracy, access, quality, humanization of care and social control. The 12th national conference, in 2003, ushered in a third consolidation phase: 3000 delegates, 80% of them elected, and a focus on health as a right for all and a duty of the State[38].

Thailand went through similar phases. The extension of basic health care coverage by a proactive Ministry of Health, encouraged by the lobby of the Rural Doctors Association, resulted in the 1992 launch of the Decade of Health Centre Development. After the 1994 economic crisis, ministry officials started mobilizing civil society and academia around the universal coverage agenda, convening a few thousand delegates to the First Health Care Reform Forum in 1997. Liaison with the political world soon followed, with a bold move towards universal access and social protection known as the "30 Baht policy"[39]. With the National Health Act of 2007, stakeholder participation has been institutionalized through a National Health Commission that includes health professionals, civil society members and politicians.

Effective policy dialogue

The institutional capacities to enable a productive policy dialogue are not a given. They are typically weak in countries where, by choice or by default, laissez-faire dominates the approach to policy formation in health. Even in countries with mature and well-resourced health systems there is scope, and need, for more systematic and institutionalized approaches: negotiation between health authorities and professional institutions is often well established, but is much less so with other stakeholders and usually limited to discussions on resource allocation for service delivery. Policy dialogue must be built. How to do that depends very much on context and background. Experience from countries that have been able to accelerate PHC reforms suggests three common elements of effective policy dialogue:

- the importance of making information systems instrumental to PHC reform;
- systematically harnessing innovations; and
- sharing lessons on what works.

Information systems to strengthen policy dialogue

Policy dialogue on PHC reforms needs to be informed, not just by better data, but also by information obtained through a departure from traditional views on the clients, the scope and the architecture of national health information systems (Figure 5.3).

Many national health information systems that are used to inform policy can be characterized as closed administrative structures through which there is a limited flow of data on resource use, services and health status. They are often only used to a limited extent by officials at national and global level when formulating policy reforms, while little use is made of critical information that could be extracted from other tools and sources (census data, household expenditure or opinion surveys, academic institutions, NGOs, health insurance agencies, etc.), many of which are located outside the public system or even outside the health sector.

Routine data from traditional health information systems fails to respond to the rising demand for health-related information from a multitude of constituencies. Citizens need easier access to their own health records, which should inform them about the progress being made in their treatment plans and allow them to participate in decisions related to their own health and that of their families and communities. Communities and civil society organizations need better information to protect their members' health, reduce exclusion and promote equity. Health professionals need better information to improve the quality of their work, and to improve coordination and integration of services. Politicians need information on how well the health system is meeting society's goals and on how public money is being used.

Information that can be used to steer change at the policy level is quite different from the data that most conventional health information systems currently produce. There is a need to monitor what the reforms are achieving across the range of social values and the associated outcomes that are central to PHC: equity, people-centredness, protection of the health of communities and participation. That means asking questions such as:

■ is care comprehensive, integrated, continuous and effective?
■ is access guaranteed and are people aware of what they are entitled to?
■ are people protected against the economic consequences of ill-health?

■ are authorities effective in ensuring protection against exclusion from care?
■ are they effective in ensuring protection against exploitation by commercial providers?

Such questions go well beyond what can be answered by tracking health outcome indicators, resource use and service output, which is what conventional health information systems focus on. The paradigm shift required to make information systems instrumental to PHC reform is to refocus on what is holding up progress in reorienting the health system. Better identification of priority health problems and trends is important (and vital to anticipate future challenges) but, from a policy point of view, the crucial information is that which allows identification of the operational and systemic constraints. In low-income countries in particular, where planning has long been structured along epidemiological considerations, this can provide a new and dynamic basis for orienting systems development[40]. The report by the Bangladesh Health Watch on the state of the country's health workforce, for example, identified such systemic constraints and corresponding recommendations for the consideration of health authorities[41].

The multiplication of information needs and users implies that the way health information is generated, shared and used also has to evolve. This critically depends on accessibility and transparency, for example, by making all health-related information readily accessible via the Internet – as in Chile, where effective communication was considered both an outcome and a motor of their "Regime of Explicit Health Guarantees". PHC reform calls for open and collaborative models to ensure that all the best sources of data are tapped and information flows quickly to those who can translate it into appropriate action.

Open and collaborative structures, such as the "Observatories" or "Equity Gauges" offer specific models of complementing routine information

Figure 5.3 Transforming information systems into instruments for PHC reform

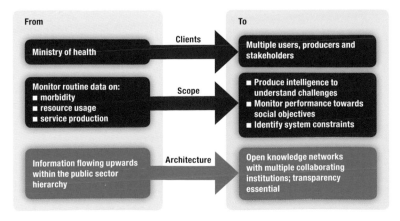

systems, by directly linking the production and dissemination of intelligence on health and social care to policy-making and to the sharing of best practices[42]. They reflect the increasing value given to cross-agency work, health inequalities and evidence-based policy-making. They bring together various constituencies, such as academia, NGOs, professional associations, corporate providers, unions, user representatives, governmental institutions and others, around a shared agenda of monitoring trends, studies, information sharing, policy development and policy dialogue (Box 5.3).

Paradoxically, these open and flexible configurations provide continuity in settings where administrative and policy continuity may be affected by a rapid turnover of decision-makers.

In the Americas, there are observatories that specifically focus on human resource issues in 22 countries. In Brazil, for example, the observatory is a network of more than a dozen participating institutions (referred to as "workstations"): university institutes, research centres and a federal office, coordinated through a secretariat based at the Ministry of Health and the Brasilia office of PAHO[44]. These networks played a key role in setting up Brazil's current PHC initiatives. Such national and sub-national structures also exist in various European countries, including France, Italy and Portugal[45]. Comparatively autonomous, such state/non-state multi-stakeholder networks can cover a wide range of issues and be sensitive to local agendas. In the United Kingdom, each regional observatory takes the lead on specific

---

Box 5.3 Equity Gauges: stakeholderholder collaboration to tackle health inequalities[43]

Equity Gauges are partnerships of multiple stakeholders that organize active monitoring and remedial action around inequity in health and health care. So far, they have been established in 12 countries on three continents. Some operate at a countrywide level, some monitor a subset of districts or provinces in a country, a few operate at a regional level and others focus specifically on equity within a city or municipality; nine have a national focus and three work at the municipal level (in Cape Town (South Africa), El Tambo (Ecuador) and Nairobi (Kenya). The Equity Gauges bring together stakeholders representing a diversity of local contexts, including parliamentarians and councillors, the media, ministries and departments of health, academic institutions, churches, traditional leaders, women's associations, community-based and nongovernmental organizations, local authority organizations and civic groups. Such a diversity of stakeholders not only encourages wide social and political investment, but also supports capacity development within countries.

Equity Gauges develop an active approach to monitoring and dealing with inequity in health and health care. They move beyond a mere description or passive monitoring of equity indicators to a set of specific actions designed to effect real and sustained change in reducing unfair disparities in health and health care. This work entails an ongoing set of strategically planned and coordinated actions that involves a range of different actors who cut across a number of different disciplines and sectors.

The Equity Gauge strategy is explicitly based on three "pillars of action". Each one is considered to be equally important and essential to a successful outcome and all three are developed in parallel:

■ research and monitoring to measure and describe inequities;
■ advocacy and public participation to promote the use of information to effect change, involving a broad range of stakeholders from civil society working together in a movement for equity;
■ community involvement to involve poor and marginalized people as active participants in decision-making rather than passive recipients of measures designed for their benefit.

The Equity Gauge strategy consists, therefore, of a set of interconnected and overlapping actions – it is not, as the name might suggest, just a set of measurements. For example, the selection of equity indicators for measurement and monitoring should take account of the views of community groups and consider what would be useful from an advocacy perspective. In turn, the advocacy pillar relies on reliable indicators developed by the measurement pillar and may involve community members or public figures.

Equity Gauges choose indicators according to the particular needs of the country as well as of the stakeholders. Emphasis is placed, however, on generating trend data within all Gauges to enable understanding of progress over time. Indicators are measured across a variety of dimensions of health, including health status; health-care financing and resource allocation; access to health care; and quality of health care (such as maternal and child health, communicable diseases and trauma). All indicators are disaggregated according to the "PROGRESS" acronym that describes a broad range of socioeconomic factors often associated with inequities in health determinants: Place of residence, Religion, Occupation, Gender, Race/ethnicity, Education, Socioeconomic status and Social networks/capital.

issues, such as inequalities, primary care, violence and health, or the health of older people[46]. All cover a wide range of issues of regional relevance (Table 5.1): they thus institutionalize the linkages between local developments and countrywide policy-making.

Strengthening policy dialogue with innovations from the field

These links between local reality and policy-making conditions the design and implementation of PHC reforms. The build up to the introduction of Thailand's "30 Baht" universal coverage scheme provides an example of a deliberate attempt to infuse policy deliberations with learning from the field. Leaders of Thailand's reform process organized a mutually reinforcing interplay between policy development at the central level and "field model development" in the country's provinces. Health workers on the periphery and civil society organizations were given the space to develop and test innovative approaches to care delivery, to see how well they met both professional standards and community expectations (Figure 5.4). Field model development activities, which were supported by the Ministry of Health, were organized and managed at provincial level, and extensively discussed and negotiated with provincial contracts. Each province developed its own strategies to deal with its specific problems. The large amount of flexibility given to the provinces in deciding their own work programmes had the advantage of promoting ownership, fostering creativity and allowing original ideas to come forward. It also built local capacities. The downside to the high level of autonomy of the provinces was a tendency to multiply initiatives, making it difficult to evaluate the results to be fed into the policy work in a systematic way.

Table 5.1 Roles and functions of public-health observatories in England[42]

Roles	Functions[a]
Monitoring health and disease trends and highlighting areas for action	Study on the inequalities existing in coronary heart disease, together with recommendations for action[47]
Identifying gaps in health information	Study of current information sources and gaps on perinatal and infant health[48]
Advising on methods for health and health inequality impact assessment	Overview of health impact assessment[49]
Drawing together information from different sources in new ways to improve health	Health profile using housing and employment data alongside health data[50]
Carrying out projects to highlight particular health issues	A study of the dental health of five-year-olds in the Region[51]
Evaluating progress by local agencies in improving health and eliminating inequality	Baselines and trend data
Looking ahead to give early warning of future public health problems	Forum for partners to address likely future public health issues such as the ageing population and genetics

[a] Example: Northern and Yorkshire Public Health Observatory.

On balance, however, the difficulties due to the locally-driven approach were compensated for by the positive effects related to reform dynamics and capacity building. By 2001, nearly half of Thailand's 76 provinces were experimenting with organizational innovation, most of it around issues of equitable access, local health-care systems and community health[52].

Thailand's "30 Baht" universal coverage reform was a bold political initiative to improve health equity. Its transformation into a concrete reality was made possible through the accumulated experience from the field and through the alliances the fieldwork had built between health workers, civil society organizations and the public. When the scheme was launched in 2001, these provinces were ready to pilot and implement the

Figure 5.4 Mutual reinforcement between innovation in the field and policy development in the health reform process

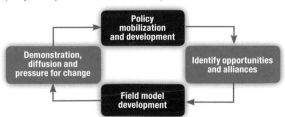

scheme. Furthermore, the organizational models they had developed informed the translation of political commitment to universal coverage into concrete measures and regulations[53].

This mutually reinforcing process of linking policy development with learning from the field is important for several reasons:

■ it taps the wealth of latent knowledge and innovation within the health sector;

■ bold experiments in the field give front-line workers, system leaders and the public an inspiring glimpse of what the future might look like in a health system shaped by PHC values. This overcomes one of the greatest obstacles to bold change in systems – people's inability to imagine that things could actually be different and be an opportunity rather than a threat;

■ the linking of policy development with front-line action fosters alliances and support from within the sector, without which far-reaching reform is not sustainable;

■ such processes engage society both locally and at national level, generating the demand for change that is essential in building political commitment and maintaining the momentum for reform.

Building a critical mass of capacity for change

The stimulation of open, collaborative structures that supply reforms with strategic intelligence and harness innovation throughout the health system requires a critical mass of committed and experienced people and institutions. They must not only carry out technical and organizational tasks, but they must also be able to balance flexibility and coherence, adapt to new ways of working, and build credibility and legitimacy[54].

However, that critical mass of people and institutions is often not available[31]. Institutions in low-income countries that have suffered from decades of neglect and disinvestment are of particular concern. They are often short on credibility and starved of resources, while key staff may have found more rewarding working environments with partner agencies. Poor governance complicates matters, and is compounded by international pressure for state minimalism and the disproportionate influence of the donor

community. The conventional responses to leadership capacity shortfalls in such settings, which are characterized by a heavy reliance on external technical assistance, toolkits and training, have been disappointing (Box 5.4). They need to be replaced by more systematic and sustainable approaches in order to institutionalize competencies that learn from and share experience[55].

Documented evidence of how individual and institutional policy dialogue and leadership capacities build up over time is hard to find, but a set of extensive interviews of health sector leaders in six countries shows that personal career trajectories are shaped by a combination of three decisive experiences[56].

■ At some point in their careers, all had been part of a major sectoral programme or project, particularly in the area of basic health services. Many of them refer to this as a formative experience: it is where they learned about PHC, but also where they forged a commitment and started building critical alliances and partnerships.

■ Many became involved in national planning exercises, which strengthened their capacity to generate and use information and, again, their capacity to build alliances and partnerships. Few had participated personally in major studies or surveys, but those who had, found it an opportunity to hone their skills in generating and analyzing information.

■ All indicated the importance of cooptation and coaching by their elders: "*You have to start out as a public health doctor and be noticed in one of the networks that influence decision making in MOH. After that your personal qualities and learning by doing [determine whether you'll get to be in a position of leadership].*"[56]

These personal histories of individual capacity strengthening are corroborated by more in-depth analysis of the factors that contributed to the institutional capacities for steering the health sector in these same countries. Table 5.2 shows that opportunities to learn from large-scale health-systems development programmes have contributed most, confirming the importance of hands-on engagement with the problems of the health sector in a collaborative environment.

Box 5.4 Limitations of conventional capacity building in low- and middle-income countries[55]

The development community has always tended to respond to the consequences of institutional disinvestment in low- and middle-income countries through its traditional arsenal of technical assistance and expert support, toolkits and training (Figure 5.5). From the 1980s onwards, however, it became clear that such "technical assistance" was no longer relevant[58] and the response re-invented itself as "project management units" concentrating on planning, financial management and monitoring.

The stronger health systems were able to benefit from the resources and innovation that came with projects but, in others, the picture was much more mixed. As a recurrent irritant to national authorities, accountability to funding agencies often proved stronger than commitment to national development: demonstrating project results took precedence over capacity building and long-term development[59], giving disproportionate weight to project managers at the expense of policy coherence and country leadership. In more recent years, the wish to reinforce country ownership – and changes in the way donors purchase technical assistance services – paved the way for a shift from project management to the supply of short-term expertise through external consultants. In the 1980s and early 1990s, the expertise was essentially provided by academic institutions and the in-house experts of bilateral cooperation and United Nations agencies. The increased volume of funding for technical support contributed to shifting the expertise market to freelance consultants and consultancy firms, so that expertise has become increasingly provided on a one-time basis, by technical experts whose understanding of the systemic and local political context is necessarily limited[60].

In 2006, technical cooperation constituted 41% of total overseas development aid for health. Adjusted for inflation, its volume tripled between 1999 and 2006, particularly through expansion of technical cooperation on HIV/AIDS. Adapting to the complexities of the aid architecture, experts and consultants now also increasingly act as intermediaries between countries and the donor community: harmonization has become a growth business, lack of country capacity fuelling further disempowerment.

The second mainstay response to the capacity problem has been the multiplication of planning, management and programme toolkits. These toolkits promise to solve technical problems encountered by countries while aiming for self-reliance. For all their potential, rigour and evidence base, the usefulness of toolkits in the field has often not lived up to expectations for four main reasons.

- They often underestimate the complexity of the problems they are supposed to deal with[62].
- They often rely on international expertise for their implementation, thereby defeating one of their main purposes, which is to equip countries with the ways and means to deal with their problems themselves.
- Some have not delivered the promised technical results[63] or led to unexpected untoward side-effects[64].
- The introduction of toolkits is largely supply driven and linked to institutional interests, which makes it difficult for countries to choose among the multitude of competing tools that are proposed.

The capacity-building prescription that completes the spectrum is training. Sometimes, this is part of a coherent strategy: Morocco's Ministry of Health, for example, has applied a saturation training approach similar to that of Indonesia's Ministry of Finance[65], sending out large numbers of young professionals for training in order to build up a recruitment base of qualified staff and, eventually, a critical mass of leaders. Such deliberate approaches, however, are rare. Much more common are short "hotel" training courses that mix technical objectives and exchange with implicit aims to top-up salaries and buy political goodwill. The prevailing scepticism about the usefulness of such programmes (systematic evaluation is uncommon) contrasts sharply with the resources they mobilize, at a considerable opportunity cost.

In the meantime, new markets in education, training and virtual learning are developing, while actors in low- and middle-income countries can access Internet sites on most health systems issues and establish electronic communities of practice. With contemporary information technology and globalization, traditional recipes for capacity development in poor countries are quickly becoming obsolete[54].

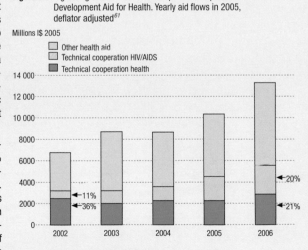

Figure 5.5 A growing market: technical cooperation as part of Official Development Aid for Health. Yearly aid flows in 2005, deflator adjusted[61]

Table 5.2 Significant factors in improving institutional capacity for health-sector governance in six countries[a,56]

Factors[b]	No. of countries where factor was an important contributor	Average score for strength of contribution
Sector programmes/ large-scale projects	4	7.25
Establishment of institutions	3	6.7
National policy debate events	3	5.6
Research, studies and situation analysis	4	5.1
New planning and management tools	1	5

[a] Burkina Faso, the Democratic Republic of the Congo, Haiti, Mali, Morocco and Tunisia.
[b] Identified through document analysis and interviews with 136 key informants.

Especially noteworthy is the fact that the introduction of tools was rarely identified as a critical input, and respondents did not highlight inputs from experts and training.

The implication is that the key investment for capacity building for PHC reforms should be to create opportunities for learning by linking individuals and institutions to ongoing reform processes. A further consideration is the importance of doing so in an environment where exchange, within and between countries, is facilitated. Unlike the conventional approaches to capacity building, exchange and exposure to the experience of others enhances self-reliance. This is not just a recipe for under-resourced and poorly performing countries. Portugal, for example, has organized a broad societal debate on its 2004–2010 National Health Plan involving a pyramid of participation platforms from local and regional to national level, and 108 substantial contributions to the plan from sources ranging from civil society and professional organizations to local governments and academia. At three critical moments in the process, international panels of experts were also invited from other countries to act as sounding boards for their policy debate: a collaboration that was a learning exercise for all parties[57].

Managing the political process: from launching reform to implementing it

PHC reforms change the balance of power within the health sector and the relationship between health and society. Success depends not only on a credible technical vision, but also on the ability to obtain the high-level political endorsement and the wider commitment that is necessary to mobilize governmental, financial and other institutional machineries.

As a technical sector, health rarely has prominence in the hierarchy of the political arena. Ministries of health have often had enough to deal with simply trying to resolve the technical challenges internal to the sector. They are traditionally ill at ease, short of leverage and ill equipped to make their case in the wider political arena, particularly in low- and low-middle-income countries.

The general lack of political influence limits the ability of health authorities, and of other stakeholders in the PHC movement, to advance the PHC agenda, especially when it challenges the interests of other constituencies. It explains the frequently absent or overly cautious reactions against the health effects of working conditions and environmental damage, or the slow implementation of regulations that may interfere with the commercial interests of the food and tobacco industry. Similarly, ambitious reform efforts are often diluted or watered down under the influence of the donor community, the pharmaceutical and the health technology industries, or the professional lobbies[26,66].

Lack of political influence also has consequences within governmental spheres. Ministries of health are in a particularly weak position in low- and low-middle-income countries, as is evidenced by the fact that they can claim only 4.5% and 1.7%, respectively, of total government expenditure (against 10% and 17.7%, respectively, in upper-middle and high-income countries)[67]. The lack of prominence of health priorities in wider development strategies, such as the Poverty Reduction Strategy Papers (PRSPs), is another illustration of that weakness[68]. Equally, ministries of health are often absent in discussions about caps on social (and health) spending, which are dominated by debates on macroeconomic stability, inflation targets or sustainable debt. It is telling that, in highly indebted countries, the health sector's efforts to obtain a share of the debt relief funds have been generally slow, less than forceful and unconvincing compared to education, foregoing possibilities for rapid expansion of their resource base[69].

Despite these challenges, there is a growing indication that the political will for ambitious reforms based on PHC is taking place. India's health missions – "rural" and subsequently "urban" – are accompanied by a doubling of public expenditure on health. China is preparing an extremely ambitious rural PHC reform that also includes a major commitment of public resources. The size and comprehensiveness of PHC-oriented reforms in Brazil, Chile, Ethiopia, the Islamic Republic of Iran, New Zealand, Thailand and many other countries, reflect very clearly that it is not unrealistic to mobilize political will. Even in extremely unfavourable circumstances, it has proven possible to gain credibility and political clout through pragmatic engagement with political and economic forces (Box 5.5).

Experience across these countries shows that political endorsement of PHC reforms critically depends on a reform programme that is formulated in terms that show its potential political dividends. To do that it has to:

- respond explicitly to rising demand as well as to the health challenges and health system constraints the country faces, showing that it is not merely a technical programme, but one rooted in concerns relevant to society;
- specify the expected health, social and political returns, as well as the relevant costs, in order to demonstrate the expected political mileage as well as its affordability;
- be visibly based on the key constituencies' consensus to tackle the obstacles to PHC, providing reassurance of the reforms' political feasibility.

Creating the political alignment and commitment to reform, however, is only a first step. Insufficient preparation of its implementation is often the weak point. Of particular importance is an understanding of resistance to change,

particularly from health workers[70,71,72,73]. While the intuition of leadership has its merits, it is also possible to organize more systematic exercises to anticipate and respond to the potential reactions of stakeholders and the public: political mapping exercises, as in Lebanon[34]; marketing studies and opinion polls, as in the United States[74]; public hearings, as in Canada; or sector-wide meetings of stakeholders, as in the *Etats Généraux de la Santé* in French-speaking Africa. Delivering on PHC reforms requires a sustained management capacity across levels of the system, embedded in institutions that are fit for the purpose. In Chile, for example, administrative structures and competencies across the whole of the Ministry of Health are being redefined in line with the PHC reforms. Such structural changes are not sufficient. They need to be instigated in conjunction with changes in the organizational culture, from one of issuing decrees for change to a more inclusive collaboration with a variety of stakeholders across the levels of the health system. That in turn requires the institutionalization of policy-dialogue mechanisms drawing practice-based knowledge up from the ground level to inform overall systems governance, while reinforcing social linkages and collaborative action among constituencies at community level[75]. This management capacity should not be assumed, it requires active investment.

Even with effective political dialogue to gain consensus on specific PHC reforms and the requisite management for implementation across levels of the system, many such reforms do not have their intended impact. The best-planned and executed policy reforms often run into unanticipated challenges or rapidly changing contexts. Broad experience in dealing with complex systems behaviour suggests that significant shortfalls or shifts away from articulated goals are to be expected. An important component to build into the reform processes is mechanisms that can pick up significant unintended consequences or deviations from expected performance benchmarks, which allow for course corrections during implementation.

Widespread evidence on inequities in health and health care in virtually all countries is a humbling reminder of the difficulties confronting

Box 5.5 Rebuilding leadership in health in the aftermath of war and economic collapse

Recent developments in the Democratic Republic of the Congo show how renewed leadership can emerge even under extremely challenging conditions. The beginnings of the reconstruction of the country's health system, devastated by economic collapse and state failure culminating in a brutal war is, above all, a story of skilful political management.

The Democratic Republic of the Congo had seen a number of successful experiences in PHC development at the district level during the 1970s and early 1980s. The economic and political turmoil from the mid-1980s onwards saw central government authority in health disintegrate, with an extreme pauperization of the health system and the workers within it. Health workers developed a multiplicity of survival strategies, charging patients and capitalizing on the many aid-funded projects, with little regard for the consequences for the health system. Donors and international partners lost confidence in the district model of integrated service delivery in the country and instead chose to back stand-alone disease control and humanitarian aid programmes. While, between 1999 and 2002, the Ministry of Health commanded less than 0.5% of total government expenditure, its central administration and its Department of Planning and Studies – 15 staff in total – faced the overwhelming task of providing guidance to some 25 bilateral and multilateral agencies, more than 60 international and 200 national NGOs, 53 disease control programmes (with 13 government donor coordination committees) and 13 provincial ministries of health – not forgetting health-care structures organized by private companies and universities.

As the intensity of civil strife abated, a number of key Ministry of Health staff took it upon themselves to revitalize and update the district model of primary health care. Aware of the marginal position of the Ministry in the health sector, they co-opted the "internal diaspora" (former civil servants now working for the many international development agencies present in the country) in an open structure around the Ministry. This steering group drafted a national health systems strengthening strategy. It included (i) a progressive roll-out of integrated services, district by district, coordinated through regional plans and backed by a fundamental shift in funding from programme-specific flows to system funding; (ii) a set of protective "damage-control" measures to halt institutional inflation and prevent further distortion of the system; and (iii) an explicit plan to tackle the problem of donor fragmentation, which had reached critical proportions. In designing the strategy, the steering group made deliberate efforts to set up networks within the health sector itself and alliances with other government actors and social constituencies.

The formal endorsement of the national plan by donors and civil society sent a strong political signal of the success of this new mode of working. The national health systems strengthening strategy became the health component of the national poverty reduction strategy. Donors and international partners aligned existing projects, albeit to a variable degree, while others reshaped new initiatives to fit the national strategy.

Perhaps the most powerful testimony to the effective management of this process is the change in the composition of donor funding for health (Figure 5.6). The proportion of funds dedicated to general systems strengthening under provincial and district plans has increased appreciably in relation to the level of funding earmarked for disease control and humanitarian relief programmes. The advances remain fragile, in a context where much of the health sector – including its governance – needs to be reconstructed.

Nevertheless, the national strategy has strong roots in fieldwork and, in a remarkable turnaround against high odds, the Ministry of Health has gained credibility with other stakeholders and has improved its position in renegotiating the finances of the health sector.

Figure 5.6 Re-emerging national leadership in health: the shift in donor funding towards integrated health systems support, and its impact on the Democratic Republic of the Congo's 2004 PHC strategy

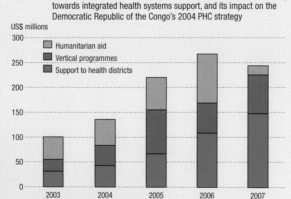

US$ millions

Humanitarian aid
Vertical programmes
Support to health districts

PHC reforms. This chapter has emphasized that leadership for greater equity in health must be an effort undertaken by the whole of society and engage all relevant stakeholders. Mediating multi-stakeholder dialogues around ambitious reforms be they for universal coverage or primary care places a high premium on effective government. This requires re-orienting information systems the better to inform and evaluate reforms, building field-based innovations into the design and redesign of reforms, and drawing on experienced and committed individuals to manage the direction and implementation of reforms. While not a recipe, these elements of leadership and effective government constitute in and of themselves a major focus of reform for PHC. Without reforms in leadership and effective government, other PHC reforms are very unlikely to succeed. While necessary, therefore, they are not sufficient conditions for PHC reforms to succeed. The next chapter describes how the four sets of PHC reforms must be adapted to vastly different national contexts while mobilizing a common set of drivers to advance equity in health.

References

1. Porter D. *Health, civilization and the state. A history of public health from ancient to modern times*. London and New York, Routledge, 1999.
2. *The World Health Report 2000 – Health systems: improving performance*. Geneva, World Health Organization, 2000.
3. Waldman R. *Health programming for rebuilding states: a briefing paper*. Arlington VA, Partnership for Child Health Care, Basic Support for Institutionalizing Child Survival (BASICS), 2007.
4. *National health accounts*. Geneva, World Health Organization (http://www.who.int/nha/country/en/index.html, accessed May 2008).
5. Schoen C et al. US health system performance: a national scorecard. *Health Affairs*, 2006, 25(Web Exclusive):w457–w475.
6. Jacobs LR, Shapiro RY. Public opinion's tilt against private enterprise. *Health Affairs*, 1994, 13:285–289.
7. Blendon RJ, Menson JM. Americans' views on health policy: a fifty year historical perspective. *Health Affairs*, 2001, 20:33–46.
8. Fox DM. The medical institutions and the state. In: Bynum WF, Porter R, eds. *Companion encyclopedia of the history of medicine*. London and New York, Routledge, 1993, 50:1204–1230.
9. Blank RH. *The price of life: the future of American health care*. New York NY, Colombia University Press, 1997.
10. Frenk J, Donabedian A. State intervention in health care: type, trends and determinants. *Health Policy and Planning*, 1987, 2:17–31.
11. Blumenthal D, Hsiao W. Privatization and its discontents – the evolving Chinese health care system. *New England Journal of Medicine*, 2005, 353:1165–1170.
12. Liu Y, Hsiao WC, Eggleston K. Equity in health and health care: the Chinese experience. *Social Science and Medicine*, 1999, 49:1349–1356.
13. Bloom G, Xingyuan G. Health sector reform: lessons from China. *Social Science and Medicine*, 1997, 45:351–360.
14. Tang S, Cheng X, Xu L. *Urban social health insurance in China*. Eschborn, Gesellschaft für Technische Zusammenarbeit and International Labour Organization, 2007.
15. China: long-term issues and options in the health transition. Washington DC, The World Bank, 1992.
16. China statistics 2007. Beijing, Ministry of Health, 2007 (http://moh.gov.cn/open/statistics/year2007/p83.htm, accessed 31 May 2008).
17. *WHO mortality database*. Geneva, World Health Organization, 2007 (Tables; http://www.who.int/healthinfo/mortdbases/en/indcx.html, accessed 1 July 2008).
18. Suhrcke M, Rocco L, McKee M. *Health: a vital investment for economic development in eastern Europe and central Asia*. Copenhagen, World Health Organization Regional Office for Europe, European Observatory on Health Systems and Policies (http://www.euro.who.int/observatory/Publications/20070618_1, accessed May 2008).
19. Collier P. *The bottom billion: why the poorest countries are failing and what can be done about it*. Oxford and New York NY, Oxford University Press, 2007.
20. Grindle MS. The good government imperative: human resources, organizations, and institutions. In: Grindle MS, ed. *Getting good government: capacity building in the public sectors of developing countries*. Boston MA, Harvard University Press, 1997 (Harvard Studies in International Development:3–28).
21. Hilderbrand ME, Grindle MS. Building sustainable capacity in the public sector: what can be done? In: Grindle MS, ed. *Getting good government: capacity building in the public sectors of developing countries*. Boston MA, Harvard University Press, 1997 (Harvard Studies in International Development:31–61).
22. Goldsbrough D. *Does the IMF constrain health spending in poor countries? Evidence and an agenda for action*. Washington DC, Center for Global Development, 2007.
23. Shiffman J. Has donor prioritization of HIV/AIDS displaced aid for other health issues? *Health Policy and Planning*, 2008, 23:95–100.
24. Bill and Melinda Gates Foundation and McKinsey and Company. *Global health partnerships: assessing country consequences*. Paper presented at: Third High-Level Forum on the Health MDGs, Paris, 14–15 November 2005 (http://www.hlfhealthmdgs.org/documents/GatesGHPNov2005.pdf).
25. Stein E et al, eds. *The politics of policies: economic and social progress in Latin America*. Inter-American Development Bank, David Rockefeller Center for Latin American Studies and Harvard University. Washington DC, Inter-American Development Bank, 2006.
26. Moran M. *Governing the health care state: a comparative study of the United Kingdom, the United States and Germany*. Manchester, Manchester University Press, 1999.
27. Saltman RB, Busse R. Balancing regulation and entrepreneurialism in Europe's health sector: theory and practice. In: Saltman RB, Busse R, Mossialos E, eds. *Regulating entrepreneurial behaviour in European health care systems*. Milton Keynes, Open University Press for European Observatory on Health Systems and Policies, 2002:3–52.
28. McDaniel A. Managing health care organizations: where professionalism meets complexity science. *Health Care Management Review*, 2000, 25:1.
29. World values surveys database. World Values Surveys, 2007 (V120, V121; http://www.worldvaluessurvey.com, accessed 15 October 2007).
30. Inglehart R, Welzel C. *Modernization, cultural change and democracy: the human development sequence*. Cambridge, Cambridge University Press, 2005.
31. Lopes C, Theisohn T. *Ownership, leadership, and transformation: can we do better for capacity development?* London, Earthscan, 2003.
32. Wasi P. *The triangle that moves the mountain*. Bangkok, Health Systems Research Institute, 2000.
33. McKee M, Figueras J. Setting priorities: can Britain learn from Sweden? *British Medical Journal*, 1996, 312:691–694.

34. Ammar W. *Health system and reform in Lebanon*. World Health Organization Regional Office for the Eastern Mediterranean and Ministry of Health of Lebanon. Beirut, Entreprise universitaire d'Etudes et de Publications, 2003.

35. Stewart J, Kringas P. *Change management – strategy and values. Six case studies from the Australian Public Sector*. Canberra, University of Canberra, Centre for Research in Public Sector Management (http://www.dmt.canberra.edu.au/crpsm/research/pdf/stewartkringas.pdf).

36. Chalmers I. From optimism to disillusion about commitment to transparency in the medico-industrial complex. *Journal of the Royal Society of Medicine*, 2006, 99:337–341.

37. Romanow RJ. *Building on values. The future of health care in Canada – final report*. Saskatoon, Commission on the Future of Health Care in Canada, 2002.

38. Escorel S, Arruda de Bloch R. As conferências Nacionais de Saúde na Cobnstrução do SUS. In: Trinidade Lima N et al, eds. *Saúde e democracia: história e perpsectivas do SUS*. Rio de Janeiro, Editora Fiocruz, 2005:83–120.

39. Jongudomsuk P. *Achieving universal coverage of health care in Thailand through the 30 Baht scheme*. Paper presented at: SEAMIC Conference 2001 FY, Chiang Mai, Thailand, 14–17 January 2002.

40. Galichet B et al. *Country initiatives to lift health system constraints: lessons from 49 GAVI–HSS proposals*. Geneva, World Health Organization, Department for Health System Governance and Service Delivery, 2008.

41. *The state of health in Bangladesh 2007. Health workforce in Bangladesh: who constitutes the healthcare system?* Bangladesh Health Watch (http://sph.bracu.ac.bd/bhw/, accessed June 2008).

42. Hemmings J, Wilkinson J. What is a public health observatory? *Journal of Epidemiology and Community Health*, 2003, 57:324–326.

43. Equity gauge profiles. Global Equity Gauge Alliance, 2008 (http:www.gega.org.za, accessed 24 April 2008).

44. De Campos FE, Hauck V. Networking collaboratively: the experience of the observatories of human resources in Brazil. *Cahiers de sociologie et de démographie médicales*, 2005, 45:173–208.

45. Ashton J. Public health observatories: the key to timely public health intelligence in the new century. *Journal of Epidemiology and Community Health*, 2000, 54:724–725.

46. *Intelligent health partnerships*. York, Association of Public Health Observatories, 2008 (http://www.apho.org.uk/resource/item.aspx?RID=39353 accessed 10 June 2008).

47. Robinson M, Baxter H, Wilkinson J. *Working together on coronary heart disease in Northern and Yorkshire*. Stockton-on-Tees, Northern and Yorkshire Public Health Observatory, 2001.

48. Bell R et al. *Perinatal and infant health: a scoping study*. Stockton-on-Tees, Northern and Yorkshire Public Health Observatory, 2001.

49. Grant S, Wilkinson J, Learmonth A. *An overview of health impact assessment*. Stockton-on-Tees, Northern and Yorkshire Public Health Observatory, 2001 (Occasional Paper No. 1).

50. Bailey K et al. *Towards a healthier north-east*. Stockton-on-Tees, Northern and Yorkshire Public Health Observatory, 2001.

51. Beal J, Pepper L. *The dental health of five-year-olds in the Northern and Yorkshire Region*. Stockton-on-Tees, Northern and Yorkshire Public Health Observatory, 2002.

52. *Thailand's health care reform project, 1996–2001: final report*. Bangkok, Ministry of Health, Thailand Office of Health Care Reform, 2001.

53. Tancharoensathien V, Jongudomsuk P, eds. *From policy to implementation: historical events during 2001–2004 of UC in Thailand*. Bangkok, National Health Security Office, 2005.

54. Baser H, Morgan P. *Capacity, change and performance*. Maastricht, European Centre for Development Policy Management, 2008.

55. Macq J et al. *Quality attributes and organisational options for technical support to health services system strengthening*. Background paper commissioned for the GAVI–HSS Task Team, Nairobi, August 2007.

56. Boffin N, De Brouwere V. *Capacity building strategies for strengthening the stewardship function in health systems of developing countries*. Results of an international comparative study carried out in six countries. Antwerp, Institute of Tropical Medicine, Department of Public Health, 2003 (DGOS – AIDS Impulse Programme 97203 BVO "Human resources in developing health systems").

57. Carrolo M, Ferrinho P, Perreira Miguel J (rapporteurs). *Consultation on Strategic Health Planning in Portugal*. World Health Organization/Portugal Round Table, Lisbon, July 2003. Lisbon, Direcção Geral da Saùde, 2004.

58. Forss K et al. *Evaluation of the effectiveness of technical assistance personnel*. Report to DANIDA, FINNIDA, NORAD and SIDA, 1988.

59. Fukuda-Parr S. *Capacity for development: new solutions to old problems*. New York NY, United Nations Development Programme, 2002.

60. Messian L. *Renforcement des capacités et processus de changement. Réflexions à partir de la réforme de l'administration publique en République Démocratique du Congo*. BTC Seminar on Implementing the Paris Declaration on Aid Effectiveness, Brussels, 2006.

61. OECD. StatExtracts [online database]. Paris, Organisation for Economic Co-operation and Development, 2008 (http://stats.oecd.org/WBOS/Index.aspx accessed June 2008).

62. Irwin A. Beyond the toolkits: bringing engagement into practice. In: *Engaging science: thoughts, deeds, analysis and action*. London, Wellcome Trust, 2007:50–55.

63. Rowe AK et al. How can we achieve and maintain high-quality performance of health workers in low-resource settings? *Lancet*, 2005, 366:1026–1035.

64. Blaise P, Kegels G. A realistic approach to the evaluation of the quality management movement in health care systems: a comparison between European and African contexts based on Mintzberg's organizational models. *International Journal of Health Planning and Management*, 2004, 19:337–364.

65. Lippincott DF. Saturation training: bolstering capacity in the Indonesian Ministry of Finance. In: Grindle MS, ed. *Getting good government: capacity building in the public sectors of developing countries*. Boston MA, Harvard University Press, 1997 (Harvard Studies in International Development:98–123).

66. Krause E. *Death of the guilds. professions, states and the advance of capitalism, 1930 to the present*. New Haven and London, Yale University Press, 1996.

67. *World health statistics 2008*. Geneva, World Health Organization, 2008.

68. *Poverty Reduction Strategy Papers, their significance for health: second synthesis report*. Geneva, World Health Organization, 2004 (WHO/HDP/PRSP/04.1 2004).

69. World Bank Independent Evaluation Group. *Debt relief for the poorest: an evaluation update of the HIPC Initiative*. Washington DC, The World Bank, 2006 (http://www.worldbank.org/ieg/hipc/report.html, accessed June 2008).

70. Pangu KA. Health workers' motivation in decentralised settings: waiting for better times? In: Ferrinho P, Van Lerberghe W, eds. *Providing health care under adverse conditions. Health personnel performance and individual coping strategies*. Antwerp, ITG Press, 2000:19–30.

71. Mutizwa-Mangiza D. *The impact of health sector reform on public sector health worker motivation in Zimbabwe*. Bethesda MD, Abt Associates, 1998 (Partnerships for Health Reform, Major Applied Research 5, Working Paper No. 4).

72. Wiscow C. *The effects of reforms on the health workforce*. Geneva, World Health Organization, 2005 (background paper for *The World Health Report 2006*).

73. Rigoli F, Dussault G. The interface between health sector reform and human resources in health. *Human Resources for Health*, 2003, 1:9.

74. *Road map for a health justice majority*. Oakland, CA, American Environics, 2006 (http://www.americanenvironics.com/PDF/Road_Map_for_Health_Justice_Majority_AE.pdf, accessed 1 July 2008).

75. Labra ME. Capital social y consejos de salud en Brasil. ¿Un círculo virtuoso? *Cadernos de saúde pública*, 2002, 18(Suppl. 47):55, Epub 21 January 2003.

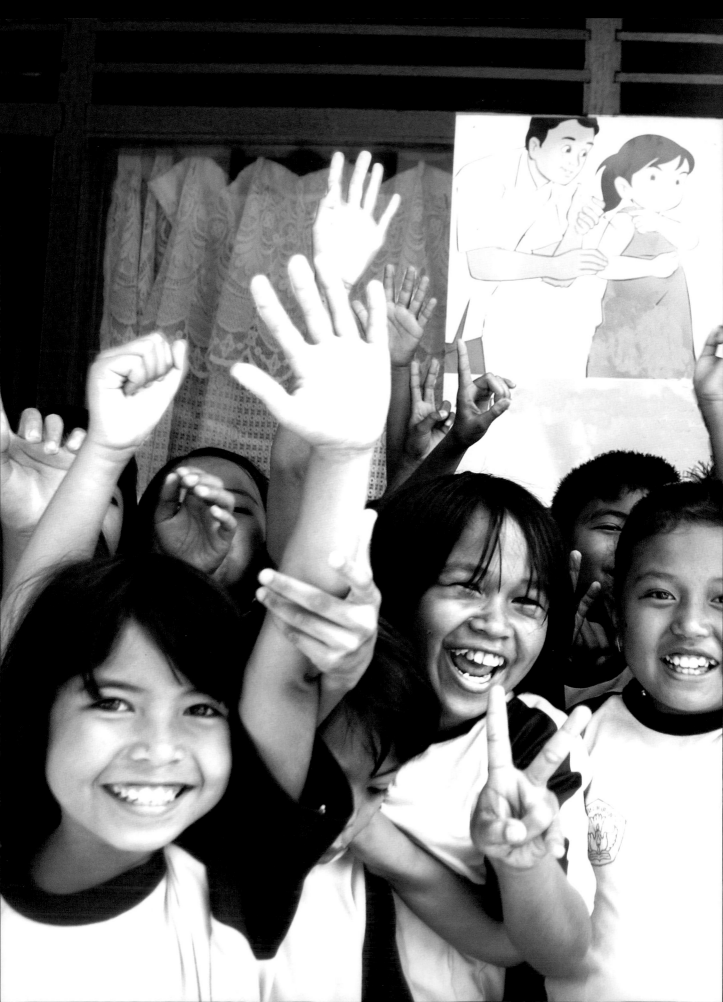

The way forward

The starkly different social, economic and health realities faced by countries must inform the way forward for primary health care. This chapter discusses the implications for the way universal coverage, primary care, public policy and leadership reforms are operationalized. It shows how expanding health systems offer opportunities for PHC reform in virtually every country. Despite the need for contextual specificity, there are cross-cutting elements in the reforms, common to all countries, which provide a basis for globally shared learning and understanding about how PHC reforms can be advanced more systematically everywhere.

Adapting reforms to country context

Although insufficiently acknowledged, the PHC movement has been a critical success in that it has contributed to the recognition of the social value of health systems, which has now taken hold in most countries in the world. This change of mindset has created a radically different health-policy landscape.

Present-day health systems are a patchwork of components, many of which may be far removed from the goals set out 30 years ago. These same health systems are converging. Driven by the demographic, financial and social pressures of modernization, they increasingly share the aims of improved health equity, people-centred care, and a better protection of the health of their populations.

However, that does not mean that health systems across the world will change overnight. Reorienting a health system is a long-term process, if only because of the long time lag to restructure the workforce[1] and because of the enormous inertia stemming from misaligned financial incentives and inadequate payment systems[2]. Given the countervailing forces and vested interests that drive health systems away from PHC values, reform requires a clear vision for the future. Many countries have understood this and are developing their strategic vision of public policies for health with a perspective of 10 to 20 years.

These visions are often couched in technical terms and are highly vulnerable to electoral cycles. Nevertheless, they are also increasingly driven by what people expect their health authorities to do: secure their health and improve access to care, protect them against catastrophic expenditure and financial exploitation, and guarantee an equitable distribution of resources[3,4]. As shown throughout this Report, the pressure that stems from these value-based expectations, if used resolutely, can ensure that the vision is not deflected and safeguard it from capture by short-term vested interests or changes in political leadership.

The protection this offers is greatly reinforced by early implementation. The possibilities to start effecting change as of now exist in virtually all countries: the growth of the health sector provides financial leverage to do so, and globalization is offering some unprecedented opportunities to make use of that leverage.

This does not in any way diminish the need to recognize the widely divergent contexts in which countries find themselves today: the nature of the health challenges they face and their wider socio-economic reality; and the degree of adaptation to challenges, the level of development and speed at which their health systems expand.

Opportunity for change is largely related to the flow of new resources into the health sector. Across the world, expenditure on health is growing: between 1995 and 2005, it almost doubled from I$ 2.6 to I$ 5.1 trillion. The rate of growth is accelerating: between 2000 and 2005, the total amount spent on health in the world increased by I$ 330 billion on average each year, against an average of I$ 197 billion in each of the five previous years. Health expenditure is growing faster than GDP and faster than population growth. The net result is that, with some exceptions, health spending per capita grows at a rate of more than 5% per year throughout the world.

This common trend in the growth in health expenditure masks a greater than 300-fold variation across countries in per capita expenditure, which ranges from less than I$ 20 per capita to well over I$ 6 000. These disparities stratify countries into three categories: high-expenditure health economies, rapid-growth health economies, and low-expenditure, low-growth health economies.

The high-expenditure health economies, not surprisingly, are those of the nearly 1 billion people living in high-income countries. In 2005, these countries spent on average I$ 3752 per capita on health, I$ 1563 per capita more than in 1995: a growth rate of 5.5% per year.

At the other extreme is a group of low-expenditure, low-growth health economies: low-income countries in Africa and South- and South-East Asia, as well as fragile states. They total 2.6 billion inhabitants who spent a mere I$ 103 per capita on health in 2005, against I$ 58 in 1995. In relative terms, these countries have seen their health expenditure per capita grow at roughly the same rate as high-expenditure countries: 5.8% each year since 1995, but, in absolute terms, the growth has been disappointingly low.

In between those two groups are the other low- and middle-income countries, those with rapid-growth health economies. The 2.9 billion inhabitants in these countries spent an average of I$ 413 per capita in 2005, more that double the I$ 189 per capita that they spent in 1995. Health expenditure in these countries has been growing at a rate of 8.1% per year.

These groups differ not only in the rate and size of their growth in health expenditure. A breakdown according to the source of growth reveals strikingly different patterns (Figure 6.1). In the low-expenditure, low-growth health economies, out-of-pocket payments account for the largest share of the growth, while in rapid-growth and high-expenditure health economies, increased government expenditure and pre-payment mechanisms dominate. Where growth in health expenditure is through pre-payment mechanisms, there is greater opportunity to support PHC reforms: collectively pooled monies are more readily re-allocated towards interventions

Figure 6.1 Contribution of general government, private pre-paid and private out-of-pocket expenditure to the yearly growth in total health expenditure per capita, percentage, weighted averages[5]

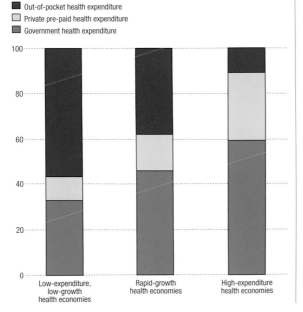

that provide a larger health return on investment than out-of-pocket payments. Conversely, countries where growth is primarily through out-of-pocket expenditures have less leverage to support PHC reforms. Alarmingly, it is in countries where expenditure is the lowest and the burden of disease highest that there is a real lack of opportunities for harnessing the growth of their health sector for PHC reforms.

The following sections outline broad categories of contexts that can shape responses for PHC reforms.

High-expenditure health economies

This group of countries funds almost 90% of its growth in health expenditure – an extra I$ 200 per capita per year in recent years – through increased government and private pre-payment funds. Expanding or changing the offer of services in these countries is less constrained by finances than by the relative lack of human resources to meet rising and changing demand. Their health systems are built around a strong and prestigious tertiary care sector that is important to the heavyweights of the pharmaceutical and medical supply industries[2]. Out-of-pocket payments, though still significant at 15% of total expenditure, have been dwarfed by more progressive collective means of financing. The third-party payment institutions have, thus, become central actors while the longstanding autonomy of the health professionals is waning. Efforts to control costs, improve quality and access to disadvantaged groups have given rise to a widening public debate on which users and special interest groups have increasing influence. Nevertheless, the state carries more weight in the health sector of these countries than ever before, with increasingly sophisticated regulatory tools and institutions.

Despite worries over their long-term sustainability, the solidarity mechanisms that finance these health systems enjoy considerable social consensus. The secular trend towards extension of coverage to all citizens, and, often reluctantly, to non-citizen residents as well, continues. In the state of Massachusetts, the United States, for example, the 2006 health insurance bill aims at 99% coverage by 2010. At the same time, it is becoming increasingly clear that universal coverage schemes need to be complemented by efforts: (i) to identify those who are excluded and set up specifically tailored programmes to include them; and (ii) to tackle the social determinants of health inequalities through policy initiatives that cut across a large number of sectors (Box 6.1), so as to translate the political commitment to health equity into concrete advances.

In many of these countries, the shift in point of gravity from tertiary and specialized care to primary care is well under way. Better information and technological developments are creating new opportunities – and a market – for moving much of the traditionally hospital-based care into local services staffed by primary-care teams or even into the hands of patients themselves. This is fuelling a change in perception of how health services should operate. It provides support for primary care, including self-care and home care. Movement in this direction, however, is held up by inertial forces stemming from the threat of downsizing and dismantling massive tertiary-care facilities and from demand induced by the illusion that the extension of life through technology is unlimited[7]. Technological innovation is indeed a driver of improvement and current trends show that it is expanding the range of services offered by primary-care teams. Technological innovation can, however, also be a driver of exclusion and inefficiency. The marked inter-country differences in the diffusion of medical technology are a reflection, not of rational evaluation, but of the incentives to providers to adopt these technologies, and the capacity to control that adoption[2].

There are two reasons why the environment in which this is taking place is changing.

- Public contestation of the management of technology has continued to increase for reasons of trust, price, exclusion or unmet need.
- Regulation increasingly depends on supranational institutions. The European Union's regulatory system, for example, plays an increasing role in the harmonization of the technical requirements for registering new medicines or of product licencing, offering possibilities, among others, for more effective support to legal provisions encouraging generic substitution for pharmaceuticals in the private sector[8]. Such mechanisms offer opportunities to increase safety and access, and thus create an environment in which national primary care reforms are encouraged.

This comes at a time when the supply of professionals willing and able to engage in primary care is under stress. In Europe, for example, the population of general practitioners is ageing rapidly, and new recruits are more likely than before to opt for part-time or low-intensity careers[1]. There is pressure to give a more pivotal role to

---

Box 6.1 Norway's national strategy to reduce social inequalities in health[6]

Norway's strategy to reduce health inequalities illustrates that there is no single solution to this complex problem. Norway has identified a large number of determinants that influence the health of individuals: income, social support, education, employment, early childhood development, healthy environments and access to health services. These complex and interrelated determinants of health are not equally distributed in society, and it is, therefore, not surprising that this leads to inequities in health as well.

The Norwegian strategy attempts to address the root causes of poor health and health inequity by influencing the underlying determinants of health, and making the distribution of these determinants more equitable from the outset. The Norwegian strategy focuses on:

- reducing social inequities;
- reducing inequities in health behaviours and access to health services;
- targeted initiatives to improve social inclusion; and
- cross-sectoral tools to promote a whole-of-government approach to health.

This brings together a number of interventions that are effective in tackling inequities, and that can be applied both within health systems, as well as through cooperation with other sectors. For instance, health systems are able to establish programmes for early childhood development as well as policies that reduce financial, geographical and social barriers to health services for those who need care the most. Working with other sectors, such as labour and finance, can create job opportunities and taxation systems that encourage more equitable distribution and redistribution of wealth, which can have a large impact on population health. In addition to universal approaches, social inclusion interventions targeted at providing better living conditions for the most disadvantaged are also critical in reducing the gaps between the most well-off and the least well-off members of society.

family physicians in primary care[9]. In the long run, however, a more pluralistic approach will be required with teams that include a variety of professionals with the instruments to provide coordination and continuity of care. That will require a different, more varied and more flexible cadre of health workers. The sustainability of primary-care reforms in the category of high-spending countries is questionable without: (i) a change in paradigm of the training of health personnel; and (ii) the necessary career, social and financial incentives to move health professionals to what in the past have been less prestigious and rewarding career options.

Spurred by the growing awareness of global health threats and of the stratification of health outcomes along social fault lines, there is a major renaissance in public health. The connections between health and other sectors are better understood and are bringing health to the attention of all sectors. Research and information systems, demand for public health training and new discourses on public health are occupying the centre stage of public concerns. This situation needs to be translated into multi-pronged cross-sector strategies to address the social determinants of health and their influence on priority health challenges (Box 6.1).

Over the last decades, most countries in this category are leading reforms through a steer-and-negotiate rather than a command-and-control approach. This reflects the growing public visibility of the health-policy agenda and the need to find a balance between the different and often irreconcilable demands of diverse constituencies. As a result, reform efforts are usually multi-levelled, with multiple actors. They progress incrementally: a protracted messy process of muddling through and hard bargaining. In England and Wales, for example, a major primary-care reform included an extensive public consultation through questionnaires addressed to more than 42 000 people, while over 1 000 individuals were invited to voice their interests and concerns in public hearings. This involvement facilitated consensus on a number of contentious parts of the reform, including shifts of resources to primary care and to underserved areas, while responsibilities were redistributed to improve cooperation and coordination[10]. Time and effort for systematic but principled negotiation is the price to pay for obtaining the social consensus that can overcome entrenched resistance to reform.

Rapid-growth health economies

In rapid-growth health economies, the challenge of engaging PHC reforms presents itself quite differently. The growing demand that comes with increased purchasing power is fuelling an expansion of services at unprecedented speed. Assuming current growth rates continue through to 2015, per capita health expenditure will grow by 60% in the fast-growing health economies of the Americas compared to 2005 levels. In the same time period, that expenditure will double in Europe and the Middle-East and triple in East Asia (Figure 6.2).

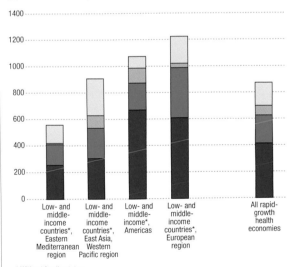

Figure 6.2 Projected per capita health expenditure in 2015, rapid-growth health economies (weighted averages)[a]

Projected total health expenditure per capita, I$, 2015
- ☐ Projected growth in out-of-pocket expenditure
- ☐ Projected growth in private pre-paid expenditure
- ■ Projected growth in government expenditure
- ■ Level of total health expenditure in 2005

* Without fragile states.
[a] Assuming the yearly growth rates for government-, private pre-paid-, and out-of-pocket expenditure estimated from 1995–2005 data[5] persist to 2015.

While the rate of growth in expenditure represents an opportunity to engage in PHC reforms, it also fuels patterns of health-sector development that run counter to the vision and values

103

of PHC. Beginnings count: policy choices that are made for political or technical expediency, such as to refrain from regulating commercial health care, may make it more difficult to redirect health systems towards PHC values at a later stage, as powerful vested interests emerge and patterns of supply-induced demand become entrenched[11]. Biases towards highly sophisticated and specialized infrastructures that cater to the expectations of a wealthy minority are being further fuelled by a new growth market in medical tourism whereby patients from high-expenditure health economies with high-fixed costs are out-sourced to these comparatively low-cost environments. This drains the supply of professionals for primary care, encouraging unprecedented rates of specialization within the workforce[12]. In contrast with these developments, ministries of health in many of these countries are still organized around specific disease control efforts, and are ill-equipped to use the leverage of expanding resources to regulate health-care delivery. The result is all too often a two-tiered system, with highly sophisticated and specialized health infrastructure that caters to expectations of a wealthy minority, in the presence of huge gaps in service availability for a large part of the population

Reforms that emphasize universal access to people-centred primary care can help to correct such distortions. These reforms can take advantage of technological innovations that facilitate rapid, simple, reliable and low-cost access to services that were previously inaccessible because they were too expensive or required complex supportive infrastructure. Such innovations include rapid diagnostic tests for HIV and gastric ulcers, better drugs that facilitate the shift from institution-based to primary care-based mental health[13], and advances in surgery that either eliminate or dramatically reduce the need for hospitalization. Combined with the multiplication of evidence-based guidelines, such innovations have considerably enlarged the problem solving capacity of primary-care teams, broadening the role of non-physician clinicians[14] and the potential of self-care. Rapid expansion of people-centred care is thus possible in a context where the technological gap between close-to-client ambulatory care and tertiary institutions is less striking

than it was 30 years ago. Chile, for example, has doubled the uptake of primary-care services in a period of five years, along with a massive investment in personnel and equipment ranging from emergency dental care and laboratories to home-based management of chronic pain. The impact of this transformation can be amplified by targeting and empowering the large numbers of poor and excluded in these countries and by reforming public policies accordingly.

In the rapid-growth health economies of the Americas and the European region less that one third of the expected growth on current trends is through increased out-of-pocket expenditure on health. Two thirds are through increased government expenditure, in combination, in the Americas, with expanded private pre-paid expenditure (Figure 6.2). The latter also plays a growing role in the Far East, where, as in the Middle East, around 40% of the growth, on current trends, will be in out-of-pocket expenditure. Leverage of PHC reforms will depend in part on the possibility to regulate and influence private pre-paid expenditure, and, particularly in Asia, to curb the reliance on out-of-pocket expenditure.

In most of these countries, the level of expenditure compared to GDP or to total government expenditure remains low, offering financial room to further accelerate PHC reforms and underpin them through parallel, and equally important, moves towards universal coverage and reduced reliance on out-of-pocket payments. In many of these countries, public resources are allocated on a capitation basis as are, at least, part of pooled private pre-payment funds. This provides opportunities to include criteria, such as relative deprivation or unmet health needs in the capitation formulas. This effectively transforms resource allocation into an instrument for promoting health equity and for introducing incentives favouring conversion towards primary care and healthier public policies.

Some of the largest countries in the world – Brazil, for example – are now seizing these kinds of opportunities on a massive scale, expanding their primary-care networks while diminishing their reliance on out-of-pocket payments[15]. Such reforms, however, rarely come about without pressure from the user's side. Chile's health policy has defined a detailed benefit package, well publicized among the population as an enforceable right. People are being informed about the kind of services, including access to specialized care, which they can claim from their primary-care teams. In combination with sustained investment, such unambiguous entitlements create a powerful dynamic for the development of primary care. Managed well, they have the potential to accelerate convergence while avoiding at least part of the distortions and inefficiencies that have plagued high-income countries in earlier years.

Low-expenditure, low-growth health economies

With 2.6 billion people and less than 5% of the world's health expenditure, countries in this group suffer from an absolute under-funding of their health sector, along with a disproportionally high disease burden. The persistence of high levels of maternal mortality in these countries – they claim close to 90% of all maternal deaths – is perhaps the clearest indication of the consequences of the under-funding of health on the performance of their health systems.

Worryingly, growth in health expenditure in these countries is low and highly vulnerable to their political and economic contexts. In fragile states, particularly in those located in Africa, health expenditure is not only low but barely growing at all, and 28% of this little amount of growth in recent years is accounted for by external aid. Health expenditure in the other countries of this group is growing at a stronger average rate of 6% to 7% per year. On current trends, by 2015, per capita health expenditure will have more than doubled in India compared to 2005, and increased by half elsewhere, except in fragile states (Figure 6.3). In many countries, this represents significant leverage to engage PHC reforms, particularly where the growth is through increased government expenditure or, as in Southern Africa, through other forms of prepayment. In India, however, more than 80% of the growth will, on current trends, be in out-of pocket expenditure, offering much less leverage.

Countries in these regions accumulate a set of problems that in all their diversity share many

characteristics. Whole population groups are excluded from access to quality care: because no services are available; because they are too expensive, or under-funded, under-staffed and under-equipped; or because they are fragmented and limited to a few priority programmes. Efforts to establish sound public policies that promote health and deal with determinants of ill-health are limited at best. Unregulated commercialization of both private- and public-health care is quickly becoming the norm for urban and, increasingly, for rural populations – a much bigger and more underestimated challenge to PHC's values than the verticalism that so worries the international health community.

In most of these countries, the state has had, in the past, the ambition to run the health sector on an authoritarian basis. In today's pluralistic context, with a multitude of different providers, formal and informal, public and private, only few have succeeded in switching to more appropriate steer-and-negotiate approaches. Instead, as public resources stagnated and bureaucratic mechanisms failed, laissez-faire has become the default approach to management of the health sector.

Figure 6.3 Projected per capita health expenditure in 2015, low-expenditure, low-growth health economies (weighted averages)[a]

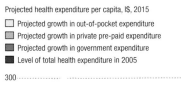

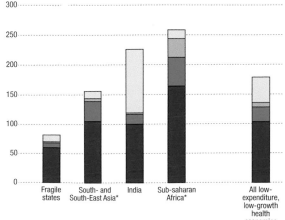

* Without fragile states.

[a] Assuming the yearly growth rates for government-, private pre-paid-, and out-of-pocket expenditure estimated from 1995–2005 data[5] persist to 2015.

This has resulted in few or feeble attempts to regulate commercial health-care provision – not only by the private, but also within the public sector, which has, in many instances, adopted the commercial practices of unregulated private care. In such settings, government capacity often limits the extent to which new resources can be leveraged for improved performance. Health authorities are, thus, left with an unfunded mandate for steering the health sector.

Therefore, growing the resource base is a priority: to refinance resource-starved health systems; to provide them with new life through PHC reforms; and to re-invest in public leadership. Prepayment systems must be nurtured now, discouraging direct levies on the sick and encouraging pooling of resources. This will make it possible to allocate limited resources more intelligently and explicitly than when health services are paid for out-of-pocket. While there is no single prescription for the type of pooling mechanism, there are greater efficiencies in larger pools: gradual merging or federation of pre-payment schemes can accelerate the build-up of regulatory capacity and accountability mechanisms[16].

In a significant number of these low-expenditure, low-growth health economies, particularly in sub-Saharan Africa and fragile states, the steep increase in external funds directed towards health through bilateral channels or through the new generation of global financing instruments has boosted the vitality of the health sector. These external funds need to be progressively re-channelled in ways that help build institutional capacity towards a longer-term goal of self-sustaining, universal coverage. In the past, the bulk of donor assistance has targeted short-term projects and programmes resulting in unnecessary delays, or even detracting from the emergence of the financing institutions required to manage universal coverage schemes. The renewed interest among donors in supporting national planning processes as part of the harmonization and alignment agenda, and the consensus that calls for universal access, represent important opportunities for scaling up investments in the institutional apparatus necessary for universal coverage. While reduced catastrophic expenditure on health care and universal access

are sufficiently strong rationales for such change in donor behaviour, the build-up of sustainable national financing capacities also offers an eventual exit strategy from donor dependence.

Governments can do more to support the health sector in these settings. Low-expenditure, low-growth health economies allocate only a small fraction of their government revenue to health. Even in sub-Saharan African countries, which have made progress and allocated an average of 8.8% of their government expenditure to health in 2005, the Abuja Declaration target of 15% is still a long way off[5]. Reaching that target would increase total health expenditure in the region by 34%. Experience of the last decade shows that it is possible to increase government revenues allocated to health rapidly. For example, following rising pressure from a broad range of civil society and political movements, India's general government expenditure on health – with a specific focus on primary health care – is expected to triple within the next five years[17]. In a different context, the Ministry of Health in Burundi quadrupled its budget between 2005 and 2007 by successfully applying for funds that became available through debt reduction under the Enhanced Heavily Indebted Poor Countries (HIPC) initiative. On average, in the 23 countries at completion point for the HIPC and Multilateral Debt Relief Initiative (MDRI), the annual savings from HIPC debt relief during the 10 years following qualification are equivalent to 70% of public spending on health at 2005 levels[18]. While only part of that money is to be directed to health, even that can make a considerable difference to the financial clout of public-health authorities.

Opportunities arise not only from increased resources. The preponderance of pilot projects is gradually being replaced by more systematic efforts to achieve universal access, albeit often for a single intervention or disease programme. These high visibility programmes, developed in relation to the MDGs, have revitalized a number of concepts that are key to people-centred care. Among them are the imperative of universal access to high quality and safe care without financial penalty, and the importance of continuity of care, and the need to understand the social, cultural and economic context in which all

---

Box 6.2 The virtuous cycle of supply of and demand for primary care

In Mali, the primary care network is made up of community-owned, community-operated primary-care centres, backed up by government-run district teams and referral units. There is a coverage plan, negotiated with the communities, which, if they so wish, can take the initiative to create a primary-care centre according to a set of criteria. The commitment is important, since the health centre will be owned and run by the community: for example, the staff of the health centre, a three to four person team led by a nurse or a family doctor, has to be employed (and financed) by the local community health association. The community can make an agreement with the Ministry of Health to obtain technical and financial support from the district-health teams, for the launch of the health centre and the supervision and back up of its subsequent operation.

The model has proved quite popular, despite the huge effort communities have had to put into the mobilization and organization of these facilities: by 2007, 826 such centres were in operation (up from 360 10 years before), set up at an average cost of US$ 17 000. The system has proved resilient and has significantly increased the production of health care: the number of curative care episodes managed by the health centres has been multiplied by 2.1. The number of women followed up in antenatal care has been multiplied by 2.7 and births attended by a health professional by 2.5, with coverage levels as measured through Demographic Health Surveys in 2006 standing at 70% and 49%, respectively; DTP3 vaccination coverage in 2006 was 68%.

People obviously consider the investment worthwhile. Twice during the last 10 years, between 2000 and 2001 and 2004 and 2005, demand and local initiative for the creation of new centres was rising so fast that Mali's health authorities had to take measures to slow down the expansion of the network in order to be able to guarantee quality standards (Figure 6.4). This suggests that the virtuous cycle of increased demand and improved

Figure 6.4 The progressive extension of coverage by community-owned, community–operated health centres in Mali, 1998–2007

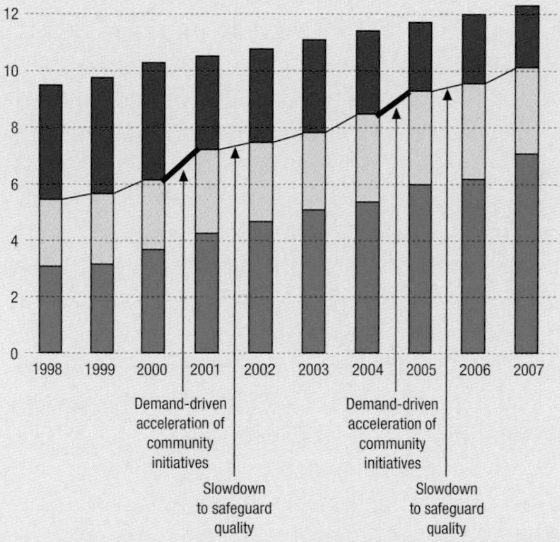

Population (millions)
- ■ Not yet covered
- □ Covered, but living more than 5 km from health care
- ▨ Covered, living within 5 km of health care

Source: Système national d'information sanitaire (SNIS), Cellule de Planification et de Statistiques Ministère de la Santé Mali [National health information system (SNIS), Planning and Statistics Unit, Ministry of Health, Mali].

supply is functioning. Health authorities are expanding the range of services offered and improving the quality – by encouraging the recruitment of doctors in the rural primary-care centres – while continuing their support to the extension of the network.

---

men, women and families of a given community live. Integration is becoming a reality through approaches, such as the Integrated Management of Adolescent and Adult Illness (IMAI) and the community-based interventions emerging from the Onchocerciasis Control Programme (OCP)[19]. Global initiatives are loosening their grip on disease-control mandates and are beginning to appreciate the importance of strengthening the system more generally, such as through GAVI Alliance's Health System Strengthening window, paving the way for better alignment of previously fragmented initiatives. Driven largely by demand, information technologies to support primary care, such as electronic medical records, are spreading much faster than anticipated. Efforts to scale up HIV treatment have helped to expose the shortfalls in key systems inputs, such as the supply chain management of diagnostics and drugs, and build bridges to other sectors, such as agriculture, given the imperative of food security. Emerging awareness of the magnitude of the workforce crisis is leading to ambitious policies and programmes, including task shifting, distance learning and the innovative deployment of financial and non-financial incentives.

In this context, the challenge is no longer to do more with less, but to harness the growth in the health sector to do more with more. The unmet need in these countries is vast and making services available is still a major issue. It requires a progressive roll-out of health districts – whether through government services or by contracting NGOs, or a combination of both. Yet the complexities of contemporary health systems, particularly, but not only in urban areas, call for flexible and innovative interpretations of these organizational strategies. In many of Africa's capitals, for example, public facilities of primary, and even secondary, level have almost or completely disappeared, and have been replaced by unregulated commercial providers[20]. Creative solutions will have to build on alliances with local authorities, civil society and consumer organizations to use growing funds – pooled private pre-payment, social security contributions, funds from municipal authorities and tax-sourced funding – to create a primary-care offer that acts as a public safety net, as an alternative to unregulated commercial care, and as a signal of what trustworthy, people-centred health care can look like.

What eventually matters is the experience of patients accessing services. Trust will grow if they are welcomed and not turned away; remembered and not forgotten; seen by someone who knows them well; respected in terms of their privacy and dignity; responded to with appropriate care; informed about tests; and provided with drugs and not charged a fee at the point of service.

Growing trust can induce a virtuous cycle of increased demand and improved supply (Box 6.2). The gain in credibility that comes from instating such a virtuous cycle is key to gaining social and political consensus on investment in healthier public policies across sectors. Effective food security, education and rural-urban policies are critical for health and health equity: the health sector's influence on these policies depends to a large extent on its performance in providing quality primary care.

Mobilizing the drivers of reform

Across all of the diverse national contexts in which PHC reforms must find their specific expression, globalization plays a major role. It is altering the balance between international organizations, national governments, non-state actors, local and regional authorities and individual citizens.

The global health landscape is not immune to these wider changes. Over the last 30 years, the traditional nation state and multilateral architecture have been transformed. Civil society organizations have mushroomed, along with the emergence of public-private partnerships and global advocacy communities identified with specific health problems. Governmental agencies work with research consortia and consulting firms as well as with non-state transnational institutions, foundations and NGOs that operate on a global scale. National diasporas have appeared that command substantial resources and influence with remittances – about US$ 150 billion in 2005 – that dwarf overseas development aid. Illicit global networks make a business out of counterfeit drugs or toxic waste disposal, and now have the resources that allow them to capture and subvert the capacity of public agencies. Power is gravitating from national governments to international organizations and, at the same time, to sub-national entities, including a range of local and regional governments and non-governmental institutions[21].

This new and often chaotic complexity is challenging, particularly to health authorities that hesitate between ineffective and often counterproductive command and control and deleterious laissez-faire approaches to governance. However, it also offers new, common opportunities for investing in the capacity to lead and mediate the politics of reform, by mobilizing knowledge, the workforce and people.

Mobilizing the production of knowledge

PHC reforms can be spurred and kept on track by institutionalizing PHC policy reviews that mobilize organizational imagination, intelligence and ingenuity. The know-how to conduct policy reviews exists[22], but requires more explicit articulations. They need to refocus on monitoring such progress with each of the four interlocking sets of PHC reforms; on identifying, as they unfold, the technical and political obstacles to their advancement; and on providing the elements for course corrections, where necessary.

In a globalizing world, PHC policy reviews can take advantage of the emerging within- and across-country collaborative networks to build up the critical mass that can lead and implement the necessary reforms. Indeed, for many countries, it is not realistic to find, within their own institutions, all the technical expertise, contextual knowledge and necessary capacity for dispassionate analysis that PHC policy reviews require. Open, inclusive and collaborative structures, such as the Latin American observatory models[23], can go a long way in harnessing the diversity of national resources. Such models also make it possible to derive further benefits from international collaboration and to overcome the scarcities within a single nation's capacities. Policy-makers today are more open to lessons from abroad than they may have been in the past, and are using them to feed national policy dialogue with innovative approaches and better evidence of what works and what does not[22]. Embedding national institutions in regional networks that collaborate around PHC policy reviews makes it possible to pool technical competencies as well as information. Importantly, it can create regional mechanisms to get more effective representation in important but labour-intensive global bodies, with less strain on scarce national resources.

More structured and intensive inter-country collaboration around PHC policy reviews would yield better international comparative data on variations in the development of health systems based on PHC, on models of good practice and on the determinants of successful PHC reforms. Such information is currently often either absent, hard to compare or outdated. By building on networks of experts and institutions from different regions, it is possible to produce consensus-based and validated benchmarks for assessing progress and easier access to (inter)national sources of information relevant to monitoring primary care. This could make a big difference in steering PHC reforms. Various initiatives in this direction, such as the Primary Health Care Activity Monitor for Europe (PHAMEU)[24], a network of institutes and organizations from 10 European Union Member States, or the Regional Network on Equity in Health (EQUINET)[25], a network of professionals, civil society members, policy-makers, and state

officials in Southern Africa, are promising steps in that direction.

There is a huge research agenda with enormous potential to accelerate PHC reforms that requires more concerted attention (see Box 6.3). Yet, currently, the share of health expenses devoted to determining what works best – to health services research – is less that 0.1% of health expenditure in the United States, the country that spends the highest proportion (5.6%) of

---

Box 6.3. From product development to field implementation – research makes the link[27]

The WHO-based Special Programme for Research and Training in Tropical Diseases (TDR) has been a pioneer in research to inform policy and practice. TDR-sponsored studies were the first to broadly document the efficacy of insecticide-treated bednets for malaria prevention in the mid-1990s, in multi-country, multi-centre controlled trials. Following introduction of the drug Ivermectin for onchocerciasis, or "river blindness", control in the late 1980s, TDR, together with the African Programme for Onchocerciasis Control, initiated research on how best to get Ivermectin into mass distribution in the field. What evolved was a tested and fine-tuned region-wide system for "community-directed treatment" of river blindness, described as "one of the most triumphant public health campaigns ever waged in the developing world."[28]

Now, as the global health community moves away from vertical disease control, operational research is facilitating the shift. Recent TDR-supported large-scale, controlled studies involving 2.5 million people in 35 health districts in three countries have demonstrated that the community-directed treatment methods developed to combat river blindness can be utilized as a platform for integrated delivery of multiple primary health-care interventions, including bednets, malaria treatment and other basic health-care interventions, with significant increases in coverage. For example, more than twice as many children with fever received appropriate antimalarial treatment, exceeding 60% coverage on average. Critical to both the funding and execution of such research are the partnerships fostered with countries in the region, as well as other public, civil society and private institutions. The vision now is to make implementation and operations research an even more important element of global research agendas, so that new products may finally begin to yield their hoped-for health impact through sounder primary health-care system implementation. Thus, the long-standing burden of deadly diseases, such as malaria, may be more effectively addressed – through global, regional and local knowledge-sharing and cooperation.

its health expenditure on biomedical research[26]. As another striking example, only US$ 2 million out of US$ 390 million in 32 GAVI Health System Strengthening grants were allocated to research, despite encouragement to countries to do so. No other I$ 5 trillion economic sector would be happy with so little investment in research related to its core agenda: the reduction of health inequalities; the organization of people-centred care; and the development of better, more effective public policies. No other industry of that size would be satisfied with so little investment in a better understanding of what their clients expect and how they perceive performance. No other industry of that size would pay so little attention to intelligence on the political context in which it operates – the positions and strategies of key stakeholders and partners. It is time for health leaders to understand the value of investment in this area.

Mobilizing the commitment of the workforce

Each of the sets of PHC reforms emphasizes the premium placed on human resources in health. The expected skills and competencies constitute an ambitious workforce programme that requires a rethink and review of existing pedagogic approaches. The science of health equity and primary care has yet to find its central place in schools of public health. Pre-service education for the health professions is already beginning to build in shared curricular activities that emphasize problem-solving in multi-disciplinary teams, but they need to go further in preparing for the skills and attitudes that PHC requires. This includes creating opportunities for on-the-job learning across sectors through mentoring, coaching and continuing education. These and other changes to the wide array of curricula and on-the-job learning require a deliberate effort to mobilize the responsible institutional actors both within and across countries.

However, as we have learned in recent years, the content of what is learned or taught, although extremely important, is but one part of a complex of systems that governs the performance of the health workforce[1]. A set of systems issues related to the health workforce need to be guided to a

greater degree by PHC reforms. For example, health equity targets for underserved population groups will remain elusive if they do not consider how health workers can be effectively recruited and retained to work among them. Likewise, grand visions of care coordinated around the person or patient are unlikely to be translated into practice if credible career options for working in primary-care teams are not put in place. Similarly, incentives are critical complements in ensuring that individuals and institutions exercise their competencies when engaging health in all policies.

The health workforce is critical to PHC reforms. Significant investment is needed to empower health staff – from nurses to policy-makers – with the wherewithal to learn, adapt, be team players, and to combine biomedical and social perspectives, equity sensitivity and patient centredness. Without investing in their mobilization, they can be an enormous source of resistance to change, anchored to past models that are convenient, reassuring, profitable and intellectually comfortable. If, however, they can be made to see and experience that primary health care produces stimulating and gratifying work, which is socially and economically rewarding, health workers may not only come on board but also become a militant vanguard. Here again, taking advantage of the opportunities afforded by the exchange and sharing of experience offered by a globalizing world can speed up the necessary transformations.

Mobilizing the participation of people

The history of the politics of PHC reforms in the countries that have made major strides is largely unwritten. It is clear, however, that where these reforms have been successful, the endorsement of PHC by the health sector and by the political world has invariably followed on rising demand and pressure expressed by civil society. There are many examples of such demand. In Thailand, the initial efforts to mobilize civil society and politicians around an agenda of universal coverage came from within the Ministry of Health[29,30]. However, it was only when Thai reformers joined a surge in civil society pressure to improve access to care, did it become possible to take advantage of a political opportunity and launch the reform[31]. In just a few years, coverage was extended and most of the population was covered with a publicly funded primary-care system that benefit-incidence analysis shows to be pro-poor[32,33]. In Mali, the revitalization of PHC in the 1990s started with an alliance between part of the Ministry of Health and part of the donor community, which made it possible to overcome initial resistance and scepticism[34]. However, sustained extension of coverage only came about when hundreds of local "community health associations" federated in a powerful pressure group to spur the Ministry of Health and sustain political commitment[35]. In western Europe, consumer organizations have a prominent place in the discussions on health care and public policies relating to health, as have many other civil society organizations. Elsewhere, such as in Chile, the initiative has come from the political arena as part of an agenda of democratization. In India, the National Rural Health Mission came about as a result of strong pressure from civil society and the political world, while, in Bangladesh, much of the pressure for PHC comes from quasi-public NGOs[36].

There is an important lesson there: powerful allies for PHC reform are to be found within civil society. They can make the difference between a well-intentioned but short-lived attempt, and successful and sustained reform; and between a purely technical initiative, and one that is endorsed by the political world and enjoys social consensus. This is not to say that public policy should be purely demand-driven. Health authorities have to ensure that popular expectations and demand are balanced with need, technical priorities and anticipated future challenges. Health authorities committed to PHC will have to harness the dynamics of civil society pressure for change in a policy debate that is supported with evidence and information, and informed by exchange of experience with others, within and across national boundaries.

Today, it is possible to make a stronger case for health than in previous times. This is not only because of intrinsic values, such as health equity, or for the sector's contribution to economic growth – however valid they may be, these arguments are not always the most effective – but on political grounds. Health constitutes an economic sector of growing importance in itself and a feature of development and social cohesion. Reliable protection against health threats and equitable access to quality health care when needed are among the most central demands people make on their governments in advancing societies. Health has become a tangible measure of how well societies are developing and, thus, how well governments are performing their role. This constitutes a reservoir of potential strength for the sector, and is a basis for obtaining a level of commitment from society and political leadership that is commensurate with the challenges.

Economic development and the rise of a knowledge society make it likely, though not inevitable, that expectations regarding health and health systems will continue to rise – some realistic, some not, some self-serving, others balanced with concern for what is good for society at large. The increasing weight of some of the key values underlying these expectations – equity, solidarity, the centrality of people and their wish to have a say in what affects them and their health – is a long-term trend. Health systems do not naturally gravitate towards these values, hence the need for each country to make a deliberate choice when deciding the future of their health systems. It is possible not to choose PHC. In the long run, however, that option carries a huge penalty: in forfeited health benefits, impoverishing costs, in loss of trust in the health system as a whole and, ultimately, in loss of political legitimacy. Countries need to demonstrate their ability to transform their health systems in line with changing challenges as well as to rising popular expectations. That is why we need to mobilize for PHC, now more than ever.

References

1. *World Health Report 2006 – Working together for health.* Geneva, World Health Organization, 2006.

2. Ezekiel JE. The perfect storm of overutilization. *JAMA*, 2008, 299:2789–2791.

3. Halman L et al. *Changing values and beliefs in 85 countries. Trends from the values surveys from 1981 to 2004.* Leiden and Boston MA, Brill, 2008 (European Values Studies, No. 11).

4. Lübker M. *Globalization and perceptions of social inequality.* Geneva, International Labour Office, Policy Integration Department, 2004 (World Commission on the Social Dimension of Globalization, Working Paper No. 32).

5. *National health accounts.* Geneva, World Health Organization, 2008 (http//www. who.int/nha/country/en/index.html, accessed May 2008).

6. *National strategy to reduce social inequalities in health. Paper presented to the Storting.* Oslo, Norwegian Ministry of Health and Care Services, 2007 (Report No. 20 (2006–2007); http://www.regjeringen.no/en/dep/hod/Documents/regpubl/stmeld/2006-2007/Report-No-20-2006-2007-to-the-Storting.html?id=466505, accessed 19 July 2008).

7. Smith G et al. Genetic epidemiology and public health: hope, hype, and future prospects. *Lancet*, 2005, 366:1484–1498.

8. Moran M. *Governing the health care state: a comparative study of the United Kingdom, The United States and Germany.* Manchester and New York NY, Manchester University Press, 1999.

9. Heath I. A general practitioner for every person in the world. *BMJ*, 2008, 336:861.

10. Busse R, Schlette S, eds. *Focus on prevention, health and aging, and health professions.* Gütersloh, Verlag Bertelsmann Stiftung, 2007 (Health Policy Developments 7/8).

11. Rothman DJ. *Beginnings count: the technological imperative in American health care.* Oxford and New York NY, Oxford University Press, 1997.

12. *Human resources for health database.* Geneva, World Health Organization, 2008 (http://www.who.int/topics/human_resources_health/en/index.html).

13. *PHC and mental health report.* Geneva, World Health Organization, 2008 (in press).

14. Mullan F, Frehywot S. Non-physician clinicians in 47 sub-Saharan African countries. *Lancet*, 2007, 370:2158–2163.

15. World Health Statistics 2008 (http://www.who.int/whosis/en/).

16. *Achieving universal health coverage: developing the health financing system.* Geneva, World Health Organization, 2005 (Technical briefs for Policy-Makers No. 1; WHO/EIP/HSF/PB/05.01).

17. National Rural Health Mission. *Meeting people's health needs in rural areas. Framework for implementation 2005–2012.* New Delhi, Government of India, Ministry of Health and Family Welfare (http://mohfw.nic.in/NRHM/Documents/NRHM%20-%20Framework%20for%20Implementation.pdf, accessed 4 August 2008).

18. *Heavily indebted poor countries (HIPC) initiative and multilateral debt relief initiative (MDRI) – status of implementation, 28 August 2007.* Washington DC, International Monetary Fund, 2007 (http://www.imf.org/external/np/pp/2007/eng/082807.pdf, accessed 12 March 2008).

19. *Integrated community-based interventions: 2007 progress report to STAC(30).* Geneva, United Nations Development Programme/World Bank/World Health Organization Special Programme for Research and Training in Tropical Diseases, 2008 (TDR Business Line 11).

20. Grodos D. *Le district sanitaire urbain en Afrique subsaharienne. Enjeux, pratiques et politiques.* Louvain-la-Neuve, Paris, Karthala-UCL, 2004.

21. Baser H, Morgan P. *Capacity, change and performance.* Maastricht, European Centre for Development Policy Management, 2008.

22. *OECD reviews of health systems – Switzerland.* Paris, Organisation for Economic Co-operation and Development/World Health Organization, 2006.

23. De Campos FE, Hauck V. Networking collaboratively: the experience of the observatories of human resources in Brazil. *Cahiers de sociologie et de démographie médicales*, 2005, 45:173–208.

24. The PHAMEU project. Utrecht, Netherlands Institute for Health Services, 2008 (http://www.phameu.eu/).

25. EQUINET Africa. Regional Network on Equity in Health in Southern Africa, Harare, 2008 (http://www.equinetafrica.org/).

26. Hamilton M III et al. Financial anatomy of biomedical research. *JAMA*, 2005, 294:1333–1342.

27. *Community-directed interventions for major health problems in Africa: a multi-country study: final report.* Geneva, UNICEF/UNDP/World Bank/World Health Organization Special Programme for Research & Training in Tropical Diseases, 2008 (http://www.who.int/tdr/publications/publications/pdf/cdi_report_08.pdf, accessed 26 August 2008).

28. *UNESCO science report 2005.* Paris, United Nations Educational, Scientific and Cultural Organization, 2005.

29. Tancharoensathien V, Jongudomsuk P, eds. *From policy to implementation: historical events during 2001-2004 of UC in Thailand.* Bangkok, National Health Security Office, 2005.

30. Biscaia A, Conceição C, Ferrinho P. *Primary health care reforms in Portugal: equity oriented and physician driven.* Paper presented at: Organizing integrated PHC through family practice: an intercountry comparison of policy formation processes, Brussels, 8–9 October 2007.

31. Hughes D, Leethongdee S. Universal coverage in the land of smiles: lessons from Thailand's 30 Baht health reforms. *Health Affairs*, 2007, 26:999–1008.

32. Jongudomsuk P. From universal coverage of healthcare in Thailand to SHI in China: what lessons can be drawn? In: International Labour Office, Deutsche Gesellschaft für Technische Zusammenarbeit (GTZ) Gmbh, World Health Organization. *Extending social protection in health: developing countries' experiences, lessons learnt and recommendations.* Paper presented at: International Conference on Social Health Insurance in Developing Countries, Berlin, 5–7 December 2005. Eschborn, Deutsche Gesellschaft für Technische Zusammenarbeit (GTZ), 2007:155–157 (http://www2.gtz.de/dokumente/bib/07-0378.pdf, accessed 19 July 2008).

33. Tangcharoensathien V et al. *Universal coverage in Thailand: the respective roles of social health insurance and tax-based financing.* In: International Labour Office, Deutsche Gesellschaft für Technische Zusammenarbeit (GTZ) Gmbh, World Health Organization. *Extending social protection in health: developing countries' experiences, lessons learnt and recommendations.* Paper presented at: International Conference on Social Health Insurance in Developing Countries, Berlin, 5–7 December 2005. Eschborn, Deutsche Gesellschaft für Technische Zusammenarbeit (GTZ), 2007:121–131 (http://www2.gtz.de/dokumente/bib/07-0378.pdf, accessed 19 July 2008).

34. Maiga Z, Traore Nafo F, El Abassi A. *Health sector reform in Mali, 1989–1996.* Antwerp, ITG Press, 2003.

35. Balique H, Ouattara O, Ag Iknane A. Dix ans d'expérience des centres de santé communautaire au Mali, *Santé publique*, 2001, 13:35–48.

36. Chaudhury RH, Chowdhury Z. *Achieving the Millennium Development Goal on maternal mortality: Gonoshasthaya Kendra's experience in rural Bangladesh.* Dhaka, Gonoprokashani, 2007.

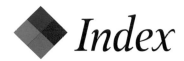

Index

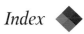